Hello, Baby!
Good-bye,
Baby Fat!

Hello, Baby! Good-bye, Baby Fat!

Sheldon Levine, M.D.

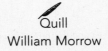

Quill
William Morrow

New York

Copyright © 1999 by Sheldon Levine, M.D.

Illustrations copyright © 1999 by Christine Leve

All rights reserved. No part of this book may be reproduced or utilized in any form or by any means, electronic or mechanical, including photocopying, recording, or by any information storage or retrieval system, without permission in writing from the Publisher. Inquiries should be addressed to Permissions Department, William Morrow and Company, Inc., 1350 Avenue of the Americas, New York, N.Y. 10019.

It is the policy of William Morrow and Company, Inc., and its imprints and affiliates, recognizing the importance of preserving what has been written, to print the books we publish on acid-free paper, and we exert our best efforts to that end.

The Library of Congress has cataloged a previous edition of this title.

Library of Congress Cataloging-in-Publication Data
Levine, Sheldon.
Hello, baby! good-bye, baby fat! / Sheldon
Levine.
p.   cm.
Includes bibliographical references and index.
ISBN 0-688-15750-5
1. Postnatal care.   2. Weight loss.   3. Puerperium—Nutritional
aspects.   I. Title.
RG801.L49   1999
618.6—dc21 98-47154
CIP

Paperback ISBN 0-688-17578-3

Printed in the United States of America

First Quill Edition 2000

1   2   3   4   5   6   7   8   9   10

www.williammorrow.com

To Richard and Ilana Rindner

and

to Arlene Ascher

For their guidance, nurturing, and love

Acknowledgments

First, thank you to a special group with whom I share something very near and dear: my last name. Janette, my wife, worked selflessly and tirelessly for long hours tightening and honing the entire manuscript. Her remarkable wit, wisdom, and devotion to the project strengthened the bonds we share each day. David and Alison made life fun as only two delightful children can. Sol and Bella managed to keep things hopping and humming along as only *they* can. Thanks for all your enthusiasm and support, Mom and Dad.

I thank Toni Sciarra, Senior Editor at William Morrow, who is a whirling dervish of ideas, energy, and vision. Her quick mind and passion for words virtually breathe a book to life. Above all, Toni remains collected even under the fire of impending deadlines. Thanks are also due to Associate Editor Katharine Cluverius, Ann Cahn, Kimberly Monroe, and Anne Nissen. Sharyn Rosenblum and her staff are wizards at public relations. I would also like to thank all of the people at William Morrow who helped with the production of the book.

Mel Berger, Vice President at the William Morris Agency, is my agent. With one "Mel-Berger look" and the widest grin imaginable, Mel speaks volumes. Speaking of volumes, the list of best-sellers he has engineered continues to mushroom, a testament to his skill and insight. And you should see him work out!

Special thanks to Brian Marks, D.C., who created the new-mom toning and back-saving plans with great care. We wish him, a chiropractor and computer consultant, and his family well as new "Tarheels." Cathy Guttman, R.D., furnished indispensable nutritional guidance by designing the menus and providing the recipes that form the nutritional backbone of the book. Cathy is a true "pro." Katy

Champ was kind enough to share some of her own engaging and delicious recipes. We look forward to her own cookbook. Jennifer Metz, fitness enthusiast and supernutritionist of tomorrow, helped buttress the nutritional science behind the recipes. Christine Leve, a talented artist, illustrated the book. She gets my trophy for her ability to pull lines and forms out of thin air.

This book is a reflection of the mountains of research materials garnered by Head Medical Librarian at the Valley Hospital, Claudia Allocco, M.L.S., and her assistant, Patrice Woods. Thank you both!

Counsel Mark Rindner provided his usual sage advice. An eternal thank-you to Betty Del Pozzo, the organizer of all good things. Sue Worth did a great job setting the bibliography straight.

One special couple came through early on by helping to clear away dark and threatening clouds of uncertainty: Dr. Ben and Vicki Co. I will never forget what you did.

Our extended family gets a big thank-you, too: Dr. Maurice and Maritta Deraney, who take such good care of our family's health and give such great tennis tips; Dr. Max and Margaret Griffel; Dr. Fred and Charlotte Reiter; Dr. Joel and Linda Moses; and Daniel and Hanka Prywes. These five couples are always first in line when it comes to giving and kindness.

John Cammarata, M.D., friend and author of *A Physician's Guide to Herbal Wellness*, advised me on all aspects of using herbs in the postpartum.

Gene Ginsburg, M.D., shared his years of experience as a gynecologist. Peter Benotti, M.D., Chief of Surgery at Englewood Hospital, is a skilled and inspiring surgeon, who teaches us that, above all, obese patients deserve to be treated with respect and dignity.

Four colleagues have made their mark by their warmth, modesty, zest, and loyalty. They are Mary Bello, M.D.; Michael Green, M.D.; Robert Port, M.D.; and Michael Scrimenti, M.D. Thank you, all.

To Chaim and Bronia Rozenblatt, thanks for a quiet summer.

The following people have all contributed, each in his or her own special way, and I thank them all. Dr. Andrew and Lori Rubin; Hal, Marti, Samantha, and David Rifkin; Ofer and Elayne Kalina; Irving and Irene Gasmer (two "tough cookies"); Dr. Jack and Debbie LeDonne; Larry and Francine Goldberg, Esq.; Dr. Mark and Susan Monane, M.S.N.; Dr. Gerard and Margaret Hansen; Bart and Ellen Gorrin; Vincent Andreano, M.D.; Megan Banta; Steve Strohlein,

M.D.; Janet Sisun; Mary Ciser; Mary Pasichnyk; Judy Lubrano; Maria Alfred; Neil and Shirley Sullivan; Larry Danziger; Fern Segal; Susan Schwarzwalder; Joan Katz; Margaret Kripackyj; Ken Goldman, M.D.; the folks at Mahwah Valley Radiology; Lois Smith; Rivka, Yehuda, and Dina Siegel; Virginia Mazza; Diane Smith; Pauline Reilly; and the great Murray Rogow. Thank you to our attorney, Jack Ballan, Esq., and his wife Sally.

Finally, to a woman of great courage, Anne Schmidt.

Contents

Part III: The Pregnancy XL Files

Part IV: The Hello, Baby! Good-bye, Baby Fat! Eating Plan

Part V: Eating in the Fast Lane

Part I

New Baby,
New Body

Chapter One

A Tale of Two New Moms

Like all doctors, I love giving people good news. But I get really excited when I have great news to share: If you are pregnant, have just delivered, or are even contemplating pregnancy, the time after delivery is *the best time ever for you to lose weight!* This is true no matter what you weigh, how old you are, how many children you have, or what your weight loss track record is.

Just ask any of the more than 10,000 women who deliver babies each day in this country. Some have gained only 15 to 20 pounds during their pregnancies; others have gained 30 to 40 pounds or more. Some are in their teens; others are in their thirties, forties, and fifties. Some are first- or second-time moms; still others already have three, four, even five or more children.

Yet less than six months after delivery, more than half of these women will weigh the same as they did before they were pregnant.

Incredibly, most of them will be back to their original shape in less than three months—some in as little as eight weeks!

Now for the real kicker. Each year 400,000 pregnant women in the United States (and millions worldwide) get the weight loss surprise of their lives: They actually lose so much weight after delivery that they weigh less than they did when they conceived! 400,000! This is not a typographical error. That's more than 1,000 women a day who defy the laws of conventional dieting by weighing *less* after birth than they did before they were pregnant. These new moms didn't only get their "old" bodies back, they got NEW, THINNER BODIES!

When interviewed, many of these women grinned and used the same expressions again and again, "The weight just seemed to come off by itself"; "My extra body fat just melted away"; or, "I really didn't do anything—the weight just flowed off me."

Obviously, something remarkable is happening to a woman's body in the period following delivery that allows for such seemingly effortless, large-scale weight loss.

The premise of this book, then, is a simple one: If indeed the body of a woman who has just delivered has unique weight loss properties (*it does!*), we should be able to identify those special properties (*we can!*) and use them so that all women who have just delivered can become the weight loss successes that they should be (*you will!*).

Hello, Baby! Good-bye, Baby Fat! shows how any woman who has recently delivered can lose both the fat she accumulated during pregnancy *and* the fat that was on her body *before* pregnancy. This new concept of weighing less after delivery than before pregnancy comes on the heels of an explosion of knowledge regarding the hormonal changes that take place in a women's body after giving birth, during the time known as the postpartum. A large number of recent medical studies reveal exciting new information that can help level the weight loss playing field for *all* new mothers, just like you. Until now, things have been far from fair. While for many women the period following birth can be the "best of times," for others it can be the "worst of times." Each year, despite their best efforts at dieting, exercising, and lifestyle changes, thousands of new moms not only have difficulty losing weight, they gain weight. And many of these women—thin before their pregnancy—"graduate" to obesity.

Why is there such a disparity in weight loss among new moms? After all, aren't the bodies of all women who have just delivered primed for weight loss? This medical paradox is best illustrated by the two women you are about to meet. Their names are Debbie and Beth, and I call their stories "A Tale of Two New Moms." They are about to give birth at any moment, so let's look in on them and see how they are doing.

Debbie's Story

It's 3:30 A.M. when Sean Jack enters the world at a hefty, healthy 8 pounds, 4 ounces, on the third floor of a community hospital in Fairfax, Virginia. The large beads of sweat that have gathered on his mother Debbie's forehead have now mixed with tears of joy streaming down her face. After a difficult seventeen hours of labor, all is well. At this moment, Debbie, a 36-year-old secretary, is not overly concerned with the 35 pounds she gained during pregnancy, though for several months now she has been eagerly awaiting the arrival of her child and the return of her waistline. Little does Debbie know that one of the first surprises of motherhood awaits her.

Over the next year Debbie will not only lose all the weight she gained while pregnant with Sean but will go on to lose the extra 15 pounds she has been carrying around for the last five years. In the end, she will weigh 130 pounds, exactly what she weighed as a college freshman, more then eight years ago! How exciting it must be for her!

Beth's Story

Just five minutes later, in a birthing room across the hall, Beth, a 27-year-old computer consultant, gives birth to a daughter, Catherine. Because the bone structure of Beth's pelvis was narrow, a cesarean section was necessary. Although she is in some pain, Beth lovingly poses with her 7-pound, 2-ounce baby as Catherine's daddy snaps away with his new digital camera. Like Debbie, Beth's weight during pregnancy reached 180 pounds. Like Debbie, weight loss is the furthest thing from Beth's mind at this glorious moment. All seems well, but there is an unforeseeable problem awaiting Beth. She will have a weight loss destiny completely different than Debbie.

Although Beth will lose 15 pounds over the next two months, after a three-month period, her weight loss will come to a complete halt. Later that year, Beth will actually gain another 10 pounds, and, as little Catherine is taking her first steps, Beth will be back at her pregnancy weight. The upward spiral will continue as she gains 2 to 3 pounds each year. Within five years she will be clinically obese, and she will have a severe weight problem for the rest of her life. To top it all off, Beth never had a weight problem before she was pregnant!

Ironically, just two days after giving birth, Beth and Debbie meet for the first time in the lobby as they prepare for discharge from the hospital. Proudly displaying their new bundles, they exchange pleasantries, then head off in different directions to start their new lives as mothers. They're also headed in two completely different directions of weight loss.

Two women, neither obese before pregnancy, both weighing the same at delivery, have completely opposite weight loss futures. Is this just a roll of the weight loss dice? A spin of the postpartum wheel of fortune?

THE GREAT WEIGHT LOSS TIME TUNNEL

No way! Something special happened to both Beth and Debbie. It is the same thing that happens to the four million women who deliver each year, and it will happen to you! It is something so obvious and straightforward that we all seem to have missed it.

Entering the period following childbirth is like entering a time tunnel of weight gain or weight loss, but exactly which direction on the scale a woman will travel has been a mystery—until now. For Beth, childbirth acted like a giant catapult, flinging her forward into the clutches of obesity. Later she would say that same terrible cliché heard around the world: "I never had a weight problem until I was pregnant."

Debbie, however, turned back the clock to the weight of her earlier years. Somehow, after delivery, Debbie overcame her body's *set point*. The set point is the weight that your body feels comfortable with and seems to rally around when you try to lose weight. It is also the all-too-familiar sticking point that heralds weight loss failure. Debbie was able to overcome her set point and reach a lower body weight—but only after childbirth. And Debbie is not alone. Each day, 1,000 women emerge from the postpartum weight time tunnel *thinner* than they were before they became pregnant. You will soon learn how you can too.

As strange as it might seem to you now, your pregnancy, along with the biochemical changes that take place in your body after delivery, are behind all this weight loss. These internal body changes will cause women like Debbie to have their own cliché, but in their case, a much happier one: "I was never this thin until I gave birth."

WEIGHT LOSS SCHOOL IS OUT FOREVER!

Some of you might be saying to yourselves, "Sure, Debbie lost all that weight; she probably did all the 'right' things: She probably exercised . . . went on a strict diet . . . maybe breast-fed." Not so. It was actually Beth, the woman who later became obese, who did all these "right" things. Beth breast-fed, joined a gym, and even hired a personal trainer. Later she tried the high-protein, high-fat diet that was the fad at the time. Soon she became desperate and starved herself on a grapefruit and rice diet. She even tried the cabbage soup diet, all to no avail.

What else could she have done? What would you have done?

THE WEIGHT LOSS MESSAGE WITHIN

One thing is certain. Losing weight after delivery is not about doing the right thing. It's not about eating less and exercising more, and it's definitely not about high-protein, high-fat diets. It's more about understanding that your body has changed in a dramatic fashion. Your internal body chemistry has made your body far too special to subject it to the usual fare of starvation diets and torturous exercise machines. Besides, what new mom has the time or energy to do all of that stuff?

It's time for you to face a whole new reality.

After nine months of weight gain, your body and brain chemistry—your hormones, enzymes, and even your metabolism—all shift naturally to help you lose weight as never before. With all of these changes taking place so suddenly, your body is sending you a weight loss wake-up call. Your body is trying to tell you that you won't be losing weight by yourself because your body will help you, once you know what you are doing. In fact, the period of time following delivery may be the first and only time in your life that your body is willing to take the lead and help you lose weight. For an overweight new mom, the stakes are higher: This might be your only chance of ever achieving a normal body weight!

That's what *Hello, Baby! Good-bye, Baby Fat!* is all about—teaching you how to listen to and understand the weight loss message from deep inside your body. This is a message that only women like you who have just delivered or are about to deliver are privy to. Go for it, just as Debbie did.

Debbie listened to her body, followed its lead, and lost all that weight—but not by following the usual diet and exercise regimens. Debbie didn't have to work that hard! Her body actually did most of the weight loss work. Beth, on the other hand, unwittingly made a few critical mistakes that put her at odds with her own body's weight loss efforts.

For starters, Beth gained far too much weight while she was pregnant. True, Beth and Debbie had the same delivery weight of 180 pounds. It's the way in which each woman arrived at this weight, though, that set the paths for their different weight loss outcomes. Debbie weighed 145 pounds at the beginning of her pregnancy, gained just 35 more with Sean, and was able to lose 50 pounds after delivery. Beth, however, started out at 125 pounds and gained 55 pounds during her pregnancy. This excess weight gain was the beginning of Beth's weight loss misfortunes.

Beth's next mistake was following a high-protein, high-fat diet in the crucial three-month period following Catherine's birth. She listened to a friend of hers who had a lost a few pounds this way. I can tell you right now (and as you'll learn in later chapters) that certain metabolic changes occur in a woman's body following delivery that make it very unlikely that high-protein or high-fat diets will work for you now, just as they didn't work for Beth.

To compound her problems, Beth began her weight loss efforts too late to allow her body to do for her what Debbie's body had done quickly and naturally. Soon you will also learn that you have a particular post-pregnancy time frame, or window, of weight loss opportunity. As the months went by, Beth's chances for weight loss diminished because her window of weight loss opportunity closed.

There is a lot that Beth could have done to slim down, but she chose a path that pitted her against her own body, sabotaging her weight loss efforts. You will learn to avoid these mistakes by putting yourself in sync with your body.

You have in your hands right now a unique weight loss plan for the unique, new you. Life with a new baby is complicated, making great demands on you both physically and mentally. Some women have jokingly told me that labor doesn't really end until they become grand-parents! Our goal is to make weight loss as easy as possible and to give each of you the chance to go beyond your pre-pregnancy weight. You will learn what works and what doesn't work. You don't need a degree in nutrition or medicine to lose weight after delivery. All you need is common sense and a scale! They will plot your course from this point on. If something makes sense and the scale goes down, use it! If not, don't!

POSTPARTUM WEIGHT LOSS MACHINES

Common sense tells us that the period following delivery, known as the *postpartum* (*post* means "after" and *partum* means "delivery" in Latin), is unlike any other period for weight loss. The average American woman gains a little over 30 pounds with each pregnancy. Approximately 20 of these pounds are composed of the weight of the baby, increased maternal tissues, and fluid. The additional 10 pounds are fat. Each pound of fat is the size and weight of a softball. In a span of just twelve to fifteen weeks postpartum, about half of all women who give birth will have succeeded in losing these 10 pounds (or more) without any great effort. That's about two million women per year. When else can so many women lose ten softballs or more of fat? In fact, as you shall see, heavier women can have even greater weight losses.

One woman I know, Elizabeth C., is a slightly built 50-year-old whom I call the "Postpartum Weight Loss Machine." She has nine children and gained 70 pounds with each pregnancy. Yet she succeeded in taking off all her weight each time, always returning to 145 pounds. This means that over the past two decades she has gained 630 pounds and lost 631. SHE ACTUALLY WEIGHS ONE POUND LESS THAN SHE DID BEFORE HER FIRST PREGNANCY!

How did she do it? Like Debbie and millions of other new moms, Elizabeth C. never knew that her new postpartum body was the result of nature's deliberate self-restoration project following the nine months of pregnancy. You never hear about such seemingly effortless weight loss in regular time—that is, when there is no pregnancy involved.

That's because 99 percent of the time your own body is unwilling to help you lose weight. After delivery, however, your body is not only ready to help you, but it leads the way!

"THE SKINNY" ON *YOUR* NEW-MOM BODY

Let's begin with a small attitude makeover.

Everyone, it seems, looks upon the postpartum as an aftermath to the joys of pregnancy. This extends to the way that women tend to view and care for their new postpartum bodies.

There is an underlying feeling in the medical community that moms should take increased care of themselves while they are pregnant, but unfortunately this level of concern drops off sharply after they deliver. An attitude like this one will never get you into those new jeans! Not a chance!

The road to the body you seek begins with a fresh new notion. The postpartum is not an aftermath. It is a new beginning.

If there is any time in your life when the majesty of your body's internal workings is evident, it is now, in the months following pregnancy. Your own body becomes your greatest weight loss ally because spectacular things are happening deep inside. Did you know that . . .

• After delivery, many of your hormones, such as estrogen, progesterone, and insulin, interact in a totally new way that suppresses your appetite.

• These hormones also fight the accumulation of any new fat deposits.

• Leptin, the newly discovered fat-burning hormone, can actually raise your metabolism and lower your set point!

• Your metabolism is higher now than it was before you were pregnant.

• You have a six- to-nine month biological clock that limits weight loss after delivery. This clock begins ticking when your baby is born.

• This biological window of weight loss opportunity has three distinct phases, each dominated by different hormones. These phases can be considered to be three new trimesters. I call them the *Three Postpartum Trimesters of Weight Loss.*

• You can put yourself in sync with the hormone pattern of each weight loss trimester through what you eat and by making small lifestyle changes specific to each trimester. We will show you how!

This is exciting stuff! You now have three trimesters of weight loss coming your way, and three different ways to lose body fat! The three postpartum trimesters of weight loss add up to this: You are now in a position not only to lose the fat that you gained *during* your pregnancy but also to lose any excess fat that you had on your body *before* you were pregnant!

Now you can begin to appreciate how special your postpartum body really is. Now you can understand why 400,000 women each year weigh less than they did before they were pregnant. Now you can begin to discover why you can say "Hello, baby! Good-bye, baby fat!"

On any given day millions of women are on diets that don't work. The reason the diets don't work is because on any given day, a woman's internal chemistry favors weight gain, not weight loss. The period of time after delivery is not "any given day." It is special, just as you are. For a few months after delivery your body will allow you to lose weight on an unprecedented scale. Think of it as a dividend from nature for nine months of "sacrificing" your body to pregnancy. Think of it as a gift.

About that six- to nine-month postpartum biological clock: Don't worry about it, because it ticks in your favor. Most of you will regain your shape and then some, much sooner than that. Studies have shown that 30 percent of new mothers need only ninety days or less to get back into their old clothes. Ninety days or less! It is comforting, though, to know that there is plenty of quality weight loss time left for larger women and for those women who have had trouble losing weight with previous pregnancies.

As a new mother, you have a lot more on your mind than weight loss. Many of you are tired, maybe even too tired to sleep. By following the weight loss plan we have laid out for you in *Hello, Baby! Good-bye, Baby Fat!*, you will not only get thinner, but you will learn which foods, vitamins, and minerals will hasten the recovery of your inner self as well. You will have more energy, sleep better, and regain the even-keel mind-set you need to enjoy the postpartum period to the fullest.

And there is even more good news. Like a good investment, losing weight after delivery also pays you a huge, lifelong health dividend.

ONE OUNCE OF PREVENTION, 30 POUNDS OF CURE

Pregnant or not, everyone, it seems, wants to lose weight. Exactly why you want to lose weight and how much weight you want to lose are very personal matters. You may want to lose weight to look better — and there is nothing wrong with that! However, weight loss after pregnancy is about a lot more than cosmetics. Weight loss after pregnancy, unlike weight loss at other times in your life, can have astonishing implications because it can prevent you from gaining weight in the future!

A major study concluded that women who retain even a few pounds after delivery stand a higher chance of becoming overweight before their next pregnancy, and obese later on. The study, published in the June 8, 1994, issue of the *Journal of the American Medical Association.* followed almost 3,000 normal-weight first-time moms. They ranged in age from 18 to 30 and came from different parts of the country: Birmingham, Alabama; Chicago, Illinois; Minneapolis, Minnesota; and Oakland, California. Five years after delivery, these new moms, despite retaining only a few pounds of their pregnancy weight, had gained on average 6 pounds more than women in the control group who were the same age and had no children. Even a small amount of retained weight after delivery put these young, healthy new mothers on a one-way street to becoming overweight.

Only now are we beginning to understand something that was known centuries ago. Ancient Greek and Chinese doctors, and later the great Islamic physicians of the twelfth century, realized that medical problems were more easily prevented than treated. Obesity is no exception. It is a lot easier to prevent weight gain than to lose weight and keep it off.

The precise reason why postpartum weight loss plays such a huge role in keeping weight off later in life is not known. Most likely it has to do with a resetting, or reprogramming of the set point that controls body weight. (We will have more to say on the subject of the set point and long-term weight control in Chapter Three.)

The latest statistics point out that 97 million Americans are either overweight or obese. That's over half of the adult population! Being overweight or obese is more common in females than males. It is felt that body differences between the sexes, including hormonal makeup, account for this gender inequality. The role that childbearing plays in skewing the number of obese on the side of women becomes clear when you consider that the average age range in which women become pregnant or obese is identical: between the ages of 25 and 44! Right now, about 35 million American women are considered obese, defined as being 20 percent above ideal body weight. You do not have to weigh 300 pounds to be obese. The average American woman is 5'4" tall and weighs 145 pounds. If you or someone you know is 5'4" in height and weighs about 175 pounds, that's more than being overweight—that's obesity!

Unfortunately, the unhealthy relationship between excess body fat and increased risk for disease is becoming all too clear. Many obese women are destined to suffer the consequences of carrying around extra fat, including heart disease (the number one killer of women), diabetes, and breast cancer. In fact, the American Heart Association recently classified obesity as a major risk factor for heart disease, ranking it right up there with smoking and high cholesterol. Lowering your weight by even 10 or 15 pounds diminishes your chances of coming down with these terrible diseases. In fact another recent study published in the *New England Journal of Medicine*, this one from Harvard University, found that women who gained more than 20 pounds after the age of 18 were two and a half times more likely to die of heart disease than women who gained less than 10 pounds. Other research found that postmenopausal women who had gained between 22 and 44 pounds were at a 61 percent higher risk for breast cancer. For many of these women, the trek toward obesity began immediately after their pregnancies. This trend crosses racial, cultural, and economic lines.

WEIGHT RELATIONS

There are a number of disturbing postpartum weight disparities you should know about. They help illustrate the true long-term importance of maximizing weight loss after delivery for everyone.

While one-third of all Caucasian adult women are obese, the percentage is far higher in the African-American and Hispanic populations. We aren't talking about being a few pounds over ideal body weight, or even about being overweight. We are talking about clinical obesity, that is, being 20 percent above ideal body weight. By this definition, more than half of all adult African-American women are obese, with the percentage being only slightly lower among Hispanic women.

Statistics show that African-American and Hispanic women not only gain more weight during their pregnancies than Caucasian women but also retain more weight after delivery. The exact reasons for these differences are unknown, but genetic, cultural, and economic factors probably play a role. The weight gain equation, however, remains unchanged. The more weight gained during pregnancy=the more weight retained after pregnancy=an increased chance for obesity later in life.

There are also definite socioeconomic issues surrounding weight loss after pregnancy. Your marital status at the time of delivery has an effect on how much you will weigh later in life. For instance, unmarried Caucasian women retain more pregnancy weight than their married counterparts. This situation is actually reversed in the African-American community. Single African-American new moms retain less weight than their married counterparts. The reason for this difference is unknown.

Your level of income is also an important indicator of your eventual postpartum weight. This reflects a larger trend found in most industrialized countries: The richer you are, the less you weigh! A pregnant woman from a household that earns less than $20,000 a year is more likely to become obese later in life.

Your level of education plays a role, too. A woman with less than one year of college education is more likely to become obese after delivery than a woman who has had two or more years of college.

Fortunately, nature is blind to race, economic, and educational status, and allows any woman to become a weight loss success after delivery. That's a great thing, because scientists have made an eye-opening weight gain projection for the United States. If obesity continues to escalate each year at the same rate as it has during the past twenty years, by the year 2150 everyone in this country will be obese! Things don't look that good for the rest of the industrialized world either. Is this the kind of unhealthy legacy we want to leave our future relatives?

Despite the opening of hundreds of new gyms, the development of thousands of new diets, and millions of weight loss dreams, the number of overweight women is rising on every continent. Despite our best treatment efforts, we now find obesity in women to be at epidemic proportions across the globe, with no relief in sight.

If our treatments for obesity are so unsuccessful, then the only solution is prevention.

The ancients were right! An ounce of prevention *is* worth a pound of cure, especially when it comes to the pounds of weight you can lose now, after delivery. Even though we don't understand why weight loss after delivery can prevent later weight gain, the fact is that it does!

If there is one time in your life when you can break the cycle of female weight gain, it is right now. So take your best shot!

Chapter Two

The "Old Wives' Tale" Club

Do you remember your literary classics from high school or college? Well, nearly all of us remember these powerful opening words of Charles Dickens's A *Tale of Two Cities:* "It was the best of times, it was the worst of times. . . . " Less well-known, though, is a later phrase: "it was the age of wisdom, it was the age of foolishness." This wonderful play on opposites just about sums up the usual approach to pregnancy and its aftermath. Explanations and attempts to understand this time of great change in a woman's life have long been steeped in folklore, old wives' tales, and, occasionally, science. Think about it: From whom did you learn about pregnancy and post-pregnancy weight loss? Your source was probably your mother, father, sister, brother, friend, or co-worker.

This is all part of the oral tradition surrounding what I call the *Mythology of Pregnancy.* Often these tales and myths contain grains of truth. Usually they are harmless, charming pieces of folklore. For example, suppose you want to conceive a boy after having given birth to two girls. You ask the womenfolk in your family for advice, and sure enough your mother-in-law chips in with this gem: For the pre-conception dinner, have a big steak (for protein), followed by a piece of Hershey's chocolate (chocolate makes you sexier). Then, after a glass of wine to change the acidity in your vagina (she's afraid to say "to loosen you up"), urinate one hour before sex. Use position number six—the one with you on top—and you will have a wonderful son just as I did." (You married him, didn't you?)

You do all of these things because, who knows, they might even work, and, more importantly, they can't hurt. Sure enough, nine months later, you give birth to a healthy boy. You then pass the formula on to your best friend Linda, who does exactly what you did. Nine months later, she gives birth to a girl! Undaunted, Linda passes the secret formula on to another friend, telling her that had she not substituted Nestlé's chocolate for Hershey's that fateful night, she, too, would have had a boy! And on and on it goes, one generation spreading the folklore of pregnancy to another.

Now, obviously this example is an exaggeration, and I'll also admit that I am guilty of spreading a few old wives' tales and "secret formulas" myself. The point is that speculation and conjecture will not get you to the level of postpartum weight loss that you need. Certainly science does not have all the answers—and it never will. However, to take advantage of the special weight loss offer that your postpartum body is making, you must be aware of the latest developments in the field.

Let's try this simple quiz to see how much you really know about weight loss after pregnancy. Answer whether the following statements are *true* or *false*:

1. Overweight pregnant women usually lose less weight after delivery than thinner pregnant women.

    ____True   ____False

2. Breast-feeding has been proved to cause weight loss after delivery.

    ____True   ____False

3. The more you exercise after giving birth, the quicker your weight loss will be.

    ____True   ____False

4. Postpartum depression is unrelated to weight loss.

    ____True   ____False

5. Return to a paying job results in increased weight loss.

    ____True   ____False

There you have it. Did you know that all of these statements are false except for one? Do you know which one is true?

Statement #1 is false. Believe it or not, overweight new moms usually lose more weight than thinner new moms. That's why the postpartum period is the overweight new mom's best chance of ever achieving a normal body weight!

Statement #2 is false. A common old wives' tale, often spread by doctors, nurses, nutritionists, and other health-care professionals, is that breast-feeding will slim down any postpartum woman in a breeze. This is simply not true. All women are different and how your weight responds to nursing depends on several factors, including genetics. Some women lose weight and some actually gain weight while breast-feeding. Learn the facts in Chapter Eight and find out what effect nursing has on your weight. You may be in for a big surprise!

Statement #3 is false. Exercise has many benefits, but frankly its role in postpartum weight loss has been disappointing. Countless old wives' tales spread by trendy magazines point to the almost limitless weight loss possibilities of exercise. Not so fast! Most studies have demonstrated that exercise has little effect on postpartum weight loss. That's terrific because most new moms are too tired and have too much to do after delivery to exercise anyway. Believe me, I was as surprised as you probably are right now when I discovered that exercise does not help the weight loss cause. Before you go out and buy that celebrity exercise video, learn the facts. *Hello, Baby! Good-bye, Baby Fat!* will show you how to become a postpartum weight loss success whether you exercise or not. In fact, what most new moms like you really need is a simple toning program to trim down those usual problem areas: the thighs, hips, and buttocks. We have it all for you.

Statement #4 is false. Contrary to popular opinion, postpartum depression is an extremely important factor in determining your postpartum weight loss success. You will learn that postpartum depression, long dismissed by the public and even health professionals as the "weepy postpartum woman syndrome" can wreak havoc not only with your self-esteem, mood, and postpartum sex life, but with your weight loss as well. Coming to grips with postpartum depression is a major factor in your eventual weight loss success.

Statement #5 is true! Women who return to work do lose more weight and lose it more quickly than those new mothers who stay at home. We will explore the fascinating mind/body connection that makes this so, and gain valuable insight into the psychological aspects of successful weight loss.

Let's look at five more old (and young) wives' tales and see how they stack up against new research.

1. **Age of Mom:** Do older new moms have more difficulty losing weight than younger ones? Decades ago, it was rare to find a new mom over the age of 30. Now the maternal age envelope has been pushed into the sixties! Although younger moms may weigh less than older moms at conception, age is *not* a factor in a woman's ability to lose weight after delivery. By the way, it was just discovered that women who conceive after age 40 have a good chance of living to 100. Right now there are 50,000 Americans above the age of 100, and most of them are women. There are a lot more to follow, because the fastest-growing sector of the American population is the age group of 80 and above!

2. **Sex of Baby:** It has been suggested that if a woman gives birth to a boy, she will lose more weight than if she had delivered a girl. Sorry, not so. In this case, there is equality of the sexes!

3. **Method of Delivery:** Many women believe that having undergone a cesarean section means more postpartum weight loss because you tend to eat less as your stomach region heals. This, too, is not true: A cesarean delivery offers no weight loss advantage over a vaginal delivery.

4. **Season of Delivery:** Part of the mythology of pregnancy maintains that women who deliver in the fall or winter retain more weight than women who deliver in the spring or summer, presumably because those women who deliver in the colder months will be less active and tend to stay indoors more. This, too, is a flight of fancy; season is no reason for weight change.

5. **Sexual Relations After Delivery:** It had been surmised that frequency of sexual relations alters postpartum hormone balance and causes a change in weight. Sorry. Weight loss is not a good reason to have, or not have, sex! (There are far better reasons, anyway!)

This is just a sampling of the new ideas that will alter the way you view both yourself and the postpartum period. Don't chain yourself to old ideas that were unhelpful in the past. The postpartum is a time of renewal. It holds out the promise of new beginnings and new possibilities, not only for your new baby but for you, the new mom.

Chapter Three

Introducing the Three Postpartum Trimesters of Weight Loss

Look at yourself in a full-length mirror. Go ahead! Face forward. How different you look! Besides the weight gain, do you notice the new-mom "glow" that everyone has been telling you about for the past few months? Look how your cheeks have filled out, nice and round! Take a half-turn and admire that new body profile. Your breasts are more ample and your protruding abdomen has reached new boundaries. Check out the new contours of your thighs and hips!

Whether you have recently delivered, or are about to, you really have changed! I hope you like what you see; after all, nature has big plans for you. To enrich your postpartum weight loss experience, it's important to understand the biochemical changes that account for the weight you have gained during pregnancy. Paradoxically, these same biochemical changes will be responsible for your reshaping after delivery.

THE MIRROR IMAGE OF YOU

What you are looking at right now in the mirror is not the real you; it is the mirror image of you—your reflection. No mirror can reflect the real you, because the real you has not changed from the outside. The real you has changed from *within*.

The changes that I am talking about are not visible in any mirror, nor to any person—including you. Ever since your positive pregnancy test, every cell inside your body has been undergoing an invisible, nine-month transformation. From the hair on your head all the way down to your toenails, every organ system has taken on the biological challenge of having another person form, develop, and grow inside of you. This all-out, all-systems effort is composed, orchestrated, and paced by a group of natural body substances located deep inside of you: your hormones.

HORMONES ARE US

Far from just being chemical messengers, your hormones are the "stuff," the very fabric, of everything about the way you look and feel. Every external change that you see in the mirror right now has an internal hormonal counterpart. The extra fat on your body is due to the action and interaction of hormones, such as estrogen, progesterone, leptin, and insulin. Your facial skin may be darker, or your hair thicker, due to increased levels of melanin and estrogen. The amount of blood in your veins and arteries increases during pregnancy, as does your heart and lung capacity, thanks to your hormones. Your metabolism rises while you are pregnant, and this too is fueled by your hormones. All the emotional highs and lows of pregnancy, delivery, and the postpartum period are induced by hormones.

You are the true star, Mom, at center stage, but hormones help run the show. It is like a wedding. The bride is the center of attention, but the caterer, the maître d', and the bandleader really make things happen.

Hormones are the caterers of your body, responsible in great part for the amount and the types of foods that you eat. Hormones have a say in every pound that you gained in pregnancy and will lose thereafter.

Hormones are also the bandleaders of your body. They are behind the way you feel about yourself and how you relate to others. But they can be two-faced like the masks of comedy and tragedy. The same hormones that make you feel so good about yourself today can bring you down to the depths of depression tomorrow. Hormones that increase your sexual desire to near-steamy levels can also make you lose interest within hours, and sometimes even within minutes. The same hormones that keep your appetite satisfied one minute can make you salivate at the sight of a hamburger commercial on TV the next minute.

These large movements of the hormonal pendulum are not due

to chance alone. These patterns are in part hereditary, which explains why you look and act more like your father than the mailman—unless, of course, the mailman is your father! It explains why you gain weight like your mother, your grandmother, or even your aunt during pregnancy, and why you tend to lose weight like them in the postpartum.

"FETAL ATTRACTION"

Whether your pregnancy test was done at home or in your doctor's office, that smile on your face and that first cry of joy were gifts from your hormones. Your pregnancy test measures the presence in your urine of a hormone, human chorionic gonadotropin, or HCG. Elevated HCG levels give the first indication that there is another person growing inside of you, one with its own life-support system: the placenta. The placenta is the organ that forms in the wall of your uterus and serves as the conduit through which nourishment passes from your body to that of your baby. The placenta also functions as a gland, manufacturing hormones. All hormones are made in glands such as the thyroid (home of the thyroid hormone), ovaries (site of estrogen and progesterone production), and pancreas (insulin). As the placenta grows and matures, it takes over many of the hormonal functions of *your* body. Not only do you have another person growing inside of you but he or she is taking control of some of *your* hormones! We could have a sci-fi movie in the making here!

Let's return to your first emotions when you learned that your pregnancy test was positive. We've noted that these intense feelings were underwritten by your hormones, including estrogen and progesterone. These hormones were aided by the "hormones of the brain," known as *neurotransmitters*.

Neurotransmitters are the natural brain chemicals that contribute to your moods, emotions, sleep patterns, appetite control, and sexual desire. These hormone-like substances, which include serotonin and dopamine, travel throughout the circuits of your brain, as well as in your blood, and are responsible for maintaining your proper mind/body connections. They help put the capital "P" in passion, but they can also put the capital "D" in depression. Being in a good mood is a reflection of these neurotransmitters working together with your hormones to keep you happy. When they malfunction, as can happen in periods of depression, stress, or fatigue, they let you down.

Pregnancy and the postpartum period bring tremendous changes in the levels of these powerful neurotransmitters. Understanding these neurotransmitters and how they work with your hormones can help alleviate the feeling that with your pregnancy, you sacrificed not only your body but your mind, too!

As your pregnancy continues, the maturing placenta develops two separate layers. The layer of the placenta that manufactures hormones makes a hormone called human chorionic somatomammotropin, or HCS. Incredible as it may seem, HCS travels through your blood and eventually reaches the appetite control center of your brain, located in the hypothalamus gland. Once there, HCS has the audacity to order your brain to increase your appetite, making you eat and eventually gain weight! This process takes place without your being aware of it. It happens within seconds, and you don't feel a thing except an increased desire to eat.

Now you understand the true meaning of why you "eat for two." You may think that you are calling all the weight-gain shots, but the reality is quite different. The little one inside is controlling *you*, using you as a shopper for and provider of all those extra calories that he or she needs to develop.

Now it's clear how so many women like Beth can say, "I never had a weight problem until I was pregnant." They're right! Pregnancy is the great hormonal appetite- and weight-booster, and you may be surprised to learn that the weight you gained during your pregnancy has a hormonal logic all its own.

THE THREE EPOCHS OF FEMALE WEIGHT GAIN

Don't think of the weight you gained during your pregnancy as just a random, chaotic, packing on of extra inches on your thighs, hips, and buttocks for the sake of your baby. Far from it! This weight gain is very carefully orchestrated and has a beautiful biological symmetry. In fact, the weight gain of pregnancy is not the isolated event it might appear to be. Instead, it is one part of a sequential weight gain trilogy that I call the *Three Epochs of Female Weight Gain*. These are three times in a woman's life when orderly weight gain is the norm. They are:

1. Puberty
2. Pregnancy
3. Menopause

Puberty signals the beginning, and menopause the end, of your ability to reproduce. On a biological time line, pregnancy, of course, fits between them. All three epochs revolve around one key element—changing levels of hormones that eventually lead to profound mind and body changes, including weight gain. In order for this to occur, your body must do one incredible, almost unthinkable thing during each epoch: It must RESET THE SET POINT!

The set point is your body's biochemical weight-control lever. Located primarily in the brain, it dictates how much weight you gain and how much you lose throughout your life. The set point can be a major obstacle to anyone attempting to reach his or her ideal body weight. Most likely each of us has more than one set point, depending upon how much we weigh. During puberty and menopause, the set point probably moves to a higher level, making you gain weight.

Working together, hormones such as estrogen, leptin, and progesterone play huge roles in the way your three epochs play out. Each epoch involves great emotional upheaval as well as weight gain, a testament to the dual mind/body roles that hormones perform. When you went through puberty, your hormones came in like a rising tide, causing your breasts to enlarge, your bones to thicken, your sexual organs to develop, and your weight to increase.

Your hormonal tide ebbs at menopause, causing the well-known thinning of bones, hot flashes, and depression, as well as changes in your heart, blood vessels, and physical stamina, and, once more, weight gain!

Pregnancy, however, is the only female weight gain epoch that is habitually followed by weight loss. This occurs because after delivery the set point lever can be pushed downward to cause weight loss. This postpartum set point quirk is the reason so many new moms like yourself are able to weigh less than they did before they were pregnant.

The weight gain of pregnancy is also the most orderly of the three epochs. While you are pregnant, nature sees to it that your weight gain hormones are introduced in phases, slowly, over nine months. Can you imagine what would happen if all your weight gain hormones intervened at the same time? You would gain all of your pregnancy weight at once — before your body had a chance to adapt. It would be like having a 30- to 50-pound weight strapped to your waist for 270 days! Imagine getting out of bed! For the next nine months you would barely be able to walk, or even breathe!

Fortunately, nature takes better care of you than that. Your weight gain follows a more gentle and logical plan. We can best understand this body logic by taking a closer look at the three trimesters of pregnancy.

THE THREE TRIMESTERS OF PREGNANCY

The notion of trimesters (from the Latin *tri*, meaning "three"; and *mens*, for "month") is a time-honored way of tracking the changes, especially weight changes, that take place in your body (and your baby's) during the nine months of pregnancy. The trimester system allows your doctor and you to track your progress until delivery and to anticipate any problems that might arise. Long before we had the technology of ultrasound, doctors had to rely on the trimester system and a scale.

The trimester system divides the nine months of pregnancy into three intervals of three months each. With the trimester system you gain perspective. When you tell people that you are in the first trimester, they know that you are in the early part of your pregnancy. Mention that you are in the third trimester, and the first thought that goes through a person's mind might be, "Hey, don't deliver here!"

The trimester system also provides a road map for weight changes that reflect the hormonal action taking place within your body. These changes are measured for better or for worse every time you get on the scale. Your weight quickly becomes a central issue of pregnancy. Almost the moment you step into the doctor's office, you get weighed. You are told how much you should weigh and how much the baby should weigh, and you are handed reams of paper about weight. Weight! Weight! Weight!

Why? Because even with the availability of sophisticated diagnostic equipment, the trimester system prevails, making your weight still the single most important monitor of a healthy pregnancy.

A typical weight gain during the nine months of pregnancy goes like this.

The First Three Months

The first trimester, or the first nine weeks of pregnancy, is characterized by little weight gain. Even after ten weeks, you might see only a 1- to 3-pound weight gain, since the placenta is still too immature to secrete the amount of hormones that will induce you to eat more. Two months after conception come alterations in the blood levels of estrogen, progesterone, leptin, and the neurotransmitter serotonin. The changing tides of these hormones are responsible not only for food cravings, but also for fatigue, nausea, sleep disturbances, breast changes, and the mood swings that characterize early pregnancy. Periods of joy and elation may be intertwined with periods of depression, weepiness, and irrational thought. Emotions are flying. Some women experience heightened sexual feelings, while others are totally turned off. If all this sounds like one big episode of premenstrual syndrome, or PMS, you are right! The first trimester is like one big PMS episode, with your body preparing itself for the arrival of your next period, which won't arrive for almost a year! But as the placenta continues to fortify itself and develop into a hormone factory, your ability to have periods departs and the stimulus to eat for two begins.

The Middle Three Months

Your real weight gain begins just prior to the second trimester. With weight gain-promoting hormones and neurotransmitters interacting at full force, an average-weight woman will gain about one pound a week during the second trimester, with her weight gain rate peaking at about the seventh month.

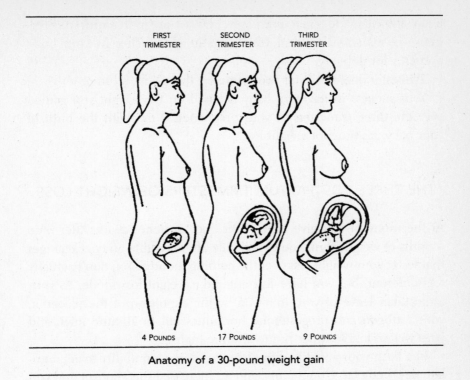

FIRST TRIMESTER   SECOND TRIMESTER   THIRD TRIMESTER

4 POUNDS   17 POUNDS   9 POUNDS

Anatomy of a 30-pound weight gain

The Last Three Months

The third trimester is almost a reverse image of the first trimester. It begins with big weight gain, which slows to a crawl before delivery. Looking at this pattern, it is apparent that the *real* weight gain of pregnancy takes place over the middle six months of pregnancy, not the full nine months.

Exceptions to this scenario are plentiful and no one follows it to a T, but in general, the weight gain that you experience parallels your baby's development. Nature is providing a slowly expanding environment in which your baby can be nurtured. In the early part of the first trimester, your placenta is small and the baby inside of you is not quite the size of a grain of rice. Nature is economizing, since at this early stage the placenta is still too immature to assimilate lots of food. The placenta, too, needs time to develop. As your baby grows and its organs mature in the second trimester, your increased food intake will ensure that it develops normally. Finally, in the third trimester, a steady state of weight gain in the fetus has been attained and great increases in food are not required. Hormone levels stabilize, and your appetite diminishes as your body prepares for delivery.

Trimester one, trimester two, trimester three—it's all so orderly!

Your success in having a baby is based on the weight you gained over the three trimesters of your pregnancy. Now, with the birth of your baby, it's time for weight loss.

THE THREE POSTPARTUM TRIMESTERS OF WEIGHT LOSS

At the moment you give birth, your body switches gears. After nine months of weight gain, you experience an incredible array of changes that foster your weight loss over the coming months. You don't actually feel different, but you have just entered a weight loss mode. As your child takes leave of you, followed by the expulsion of the placenta, your estrogen and progesterone hormones fall to all-time lows, and your weight loss fortunes rise to all-time highs.

In a flash your appetite diminishes, as does your ability to accumulate new body fat. Couple this with an increased metabolism and you have all of the ingredients for perfect, natural weight loss. I call it "natural weight loss" because it "just happens" as an act of nature. This is precisely the natural weight loss pattern that causes so many women to later say, "The weight just seemed to melt away." In fact, few women who lose a large amount of weight in the postpartum period realize how they did it or how their hormones, enzymes, and neurotransmitters all worked behind the scenes to cause this unprecedented weight loss. In the end, though, they, like you, will come to realize that their bodies were the unsung heroes behind it all. Here's how it happens.

A few days after delivery, levels of estrogen, progesterone, and some of your other hormones and neurotransmitters slowly begin to return to normal. These are the same hormones that aligned themselves so perfectly during your three trimesters of pregnancy and caused your orderly weight gain. One by one, like coats of paint, they return in precise order to pre-pregnancy levels. Your body needs your hormones to return to their normal levels in order to reestablish your menstrual cycle and provide you with the opportunity to have more babies, if you so desire. This return to biological normalcy usually takes a few months unless you breast-feed, because nursing postpones the return of regular menstrual periods.

Until your hormones function just as they did before your pregnancy, your body has a unique window of weight loss opportunity. Your hormones are now aligned in "hormone harmony"—a certain configuration that happens only once in your life: after childbirth. This new hormonal alignment makes it easier than ever for you to lose weight. How long does this grace period last? I thought you would never ask!

TIME IS ON YOUR SIDE

Your new fat-fighting, appetite-lowering hormonal changes last between six and nine months after delivery. Sound familiar? It should! In fact, it sounds like an exact reversal of the weight gain of the nine months of pregnancy.

But there is still more. A closer look at the way your hormones come back over the nine months after delivery reveals that they return in three separate phases. This, too, should sound very familiar to you. These phases are none other than three new trimesters. This time, though, with no baby on board, you lose weight during the three trimesters rather than gain weight! Your three new trimesters are based on three new and different patterns of hormones, giving you three different ways to slim down. These are your very own *Three Trimesters of Weight Loss!*

In Part II, you will be provided with the step-by-step guidance you need to navigate your *new* three trimesters, nature's own time-out for weight loss. In the meantime, here is a quick survey, or bird's-eye view, of these trimesters.

The First Trimester of Weight Loss

The first trimester of weight loss begins at delivery and lasts approximately ninety days. This weight loss trimester packs the biggest weight loss punch of the three trimesters. However, there are a few barriers to overcome, because the first weight loss trimester is dominated by immense fluctuations in both mood and energy level. The biochemical culprits include the usual suspects, estrogen and progesterone, but this time even they take a back seat to the brain hormone serotonin. Having low levels of serotonin immediately after delivery can make you depressed and put the brakes on any weight loss effort. While the body is willing, the mind is not. Watching your fat intake and increasing your intake of complex carbohydrates such as pasta, rice, and cereal can naturally raise your level of serotonin. This will, in turn, elevate your mood, give you more energy, and reestablish the all-important mind/body connection. Also, certain B vitamins and minerals play a key role in your body's attempt to restore itself after nine months of weight gain. The way you eat now will also go a long way toward getting you a good night's sleep. All told, you will not only get thinner but will feel better about yourself, too. Wearing your new happy face will enable you to enjoy the postpartum period even more.

Two major pluses of the first trimester of weight loss are an increased metabolism and a diminished appetite. You will learn how to capitalize on these biochemical quirks to further foster your weight loss. More than 30 percent of you new moms will lose *all* your pregnancy weight in the first three months, so this first weight loss trimester will also be your *last!*

The Second Trimester of Weight Loss

The second trimester of weight loss begins two to three months after delivery and is characterized by the return of your menstrual cycle. This is the most important weight loss trimester for overweight women because most of your fat will be lost during this trimester. At this point, your goal is to continue to lose weight with the help of your newly discovered fat-burning hormone, leptin (which you get to know more about in Chapter Seven). The timing is perfect because it coincides with the time that many of you will be returning to work. Just about all non-breast-feeding women will have lost most of their weight by the end of this trimester. In essence, many of you will require only two weight loss trimesters, or four to six months, to become weight loss success stories.

The Third Trimester of Weight Loss

The third trimester of weight loss begins at five to six months postpartum. This trimester is reserved for breast-feeding women who are overweight. Six months after delivery, your hormones are just about back to normal, which means that your body is no longer cooperating in the weight loss process. Only certain hormones present in an overweight, breast-feeding woman's body, as you will learn, allow her to continue losing weight at this time.

This third trimester of weight loss offers the overweight new mother a wonderful chance, and perhaps the *only* real chance, of ever attaining a healthy weight and preventing future weight gain!

Three trimesters of weight loss, three different ways that your body lets you lose weight!

"YOUR NEW MIRROR IMAGE"

At last you have discovered the true mirror image of you. Your pregnancy weight gain took place over six to nine months; now you have the same six to nine months for weight loss! This is nature showing off its symmetry and giving its reward to you for sacrificing your former shape—a shape you will now recover, and then some!

These weight loss trimesters happen to every new mom. It does not matter what you weigh or how much (or how little) you've accomplished in the weight loss arena before. There is no need for strict dieting, or for energy-robbing marathon workouts. After having a baby you have little time and energy for things like that! All you need to do is to make minimal, temporary eating and lifestyle changes that put you in sync with the hormone pattern of each weight loss trimester. This is how you amplify your own body's ability to get thinner.

My weight loss philosophy is simple. When I was a guest on *Larry King Live!*, the *Montel Williams Show, Geraldo,* and the *Today* show, I told each of the hosts what I am telling you now: I don't believe in diets! Diets are not only too restrictive but too hard to follow or swallow! Worse still, they are boring! You don't need the food police dictating what and how to eat. You are much too smart for that! What you need is a framework within which you can make your own healthy choices.

The postpartum period, with its changing weight loss trimesters, is unique in that all you need to do is make minor dieting modifications for *a few weeks* at a time. The lifestyle changes that we suggest require very little effort on your part. After all, we already said that your body does most of the work.

You had better get moving, though, because the window of weight loss opportunity does not stay open forever. Each of you has a six-month weight loss clock inside of you that begins ticking when you give birth. When the clock stops ticking, so does your weight loss, unless (as we have noted) you are an overweight woman who nurses. This concept of an internal biological clock limiting weight loss may be news to us, but it's old hat to your body.

TICK, TOCK, GOES YOUR SIX-MONTH WEIGHT LOSS CLOCK

I first learned about your postpartum six-month weight loss meter from Diane N., a 35-year-old elementary school teacher. Obese all her life, she weighed 270 pounds at the onset of pregnancy. Although she gained only 10 pounds while pregnant (because she was already so heavy), she had a difficult delivery. One week after the birth of her daughter Robin, she developed gallbladder disease and needed surgery. Diane persuaded her surgeon to perform stomach stapling at the same time she was having her gallbladder out. Stomach stapling is a surgical procedure reserved for those who are extremely obese and who have tried other methods of weight loss to no avail. The idea behind stapling is to surgically make the stomach smaller and thereby limit the amount of food and drink that the stomach can accommodate. Patients often lose huge amounts of weight by eating and drinking less after this operation.

Diane did quite well following her surgery, and after five months had lost an astounding 100 pounds! But Diane was not satisfied and wanted to lose more. She felt that after subjecting herself to such a drastic and potentially dangerous surgical procedure, she should keep going and try to reach her fantasy weight of 140 pounds (though she admitted that she would "take" 150 pounds). Despite a herculean effort, she lost just 5 more pounds over the next month, and that was it. Diane's weight loss stopped. She told me that she felt as if she had hit a brick wall. Despite consuming only 1000 calories a day, she could go no farther. This seemed very odd. Why had the stomach stapling stopped working? She should have been able to lose as much weight as she'd like, just by virtue of her stomach's being so small that it could take in only a little amount food at one time.

Then I remembered that I had seen other cases where postpartum women who had not undergone any weight loss surgery also stopped losing weight about six months after delivery. What was so daunting about six months after delivery? With this six-month time frame in mind, I reviewed patients' files to see if other postpartum women had also confronted this internal weight loss barrier. To my surprise, they had! I just had never made the connection before.

So many women like Diane, I realized, had indeed hit a wall—a biological wall much stronger than any brick wall. A further review of the medical literature revealed that just about all postpartum women have this six-month weight loss time limit, and so do you! The precise mechanism that governs this six-month barrier is not yet known. It may be due to the fact that your metabolism slows down as you lose weight, and your body adjusts to any decrease in food intake that you have made by shutting down your ability to lose weight, essentially putting your set point on hold. (Robert Nulman, a systems engineer, graphically describes this process as a "freezing" of the set point.) Therefore, the same hormones and neurotransmitters that were your postpartum allies are now your foes, once again. Nature can have some sense of humor!

There is good and bad news here. Except for overweight women who breast-feed, few of you will lose weight beyond the sixth month postpartum. The good news is that most of you will not even need six months! You will achieve weight loss success as you proceed steadily through the first few months after delivery, and you will be finished long before the six-month weight loss window slams shut.

Think of the six-month period not as a limiting factor, but rather as a gift from your body. Like the gift that Cinderella received, your gift expires, too. However, six months is a lot longer than midnight! Your body promises to be your weight loss ally for up to six months, and even longer if you are obese.

Unlike Cinderella, you aren't competing against an external mechanical clock. Yours is a biochemical clock, and after all is said and done, this clock is not only inside of you—the clock is *you!*

Go back to the mirror one more time, please, just for a moment. Think of this internal clock. Look straight ahead. There! Now you can see your own *true* mirror image.

As a reward for sacrificing your body for the past nine months, your "new" body is granting you six to nine months of postpartum weight loss. That smile on your face should be widening when you begin to realize that this weight loss gift is all yours, from your body to you!

It's like passing "Go," collecting $200, and winning weight loss Monopoly every day!

Chapter Four

The Five Factors of Postpartum Weight Loss Success

The three weight loss trimesters apply to all new moms, but the amount of weight you lose is ultimately dependent not only on the amount of energy and enthusiasm you put into your efforts, but also on five factors that can influence your weight loss outcome. I call them the *Five Factors of Postpartum Weight Loss Success*. Having most of these factors on your side will definitely facilitate your weight loss, but don't worry if you don't have all five of them. Few women do. *Hello, Baby! Good-bye, Baby Fat!* shows you how to harness the factors that you do have and make them work for you.

How did I identify these factors? They emerged from analysis of many sources, including surveys involving thousands of formerly pregnant women, discussions with weight loss experts from around the world, and, most important, extensive reviews of the latest medical literature. Decades of research have been done by major medical institutions around the world, such as Harvard University, Cambridge University, and the universities of Tokyo, Stockholm, and Madrid.

The five factors of postpartum weight loss success are based on the real-life experiences of countless women from Asia, Africa, Europe, the Americas, and Australia. We owe them all a debt of gratitude because they have taught us, in part, how to successfully navigate the three postpartum trimesters of weight loss.

THE FIVE FACTORS

1. **Utilizing Your Genetic Weight Loss Potential:** Each of you has her own obstetrical family history. Perhaps you have already noticed

that you carry and gain weight like your mother, grandmother, or sister. Like history, pregnancies tend to repeat themselves, and women will often have similar weight gains and losses with each delivery. These tendencies are not by chance; they are a by-product of your genetic makeup. Each of you has her own weight gain and weight loss potential. How well you eventually do still has roots in your family tree, and not all relatives fare the same in the genetics department.

There are three different hereditary patterns of pregnancy weight gain and postpartum weight loss. In Chapter Five you will discover what your own family pattern is, and you will learn which pattern of weight loss is best for you.

2. **Limiting the Amount of Pregnancy Weight:** As you know, there is a lot of controversy surrounding the issue of weight gain in pregnancy. Although the scientific literature suggests that the more weight is gained during pregnancy, the more weight is retained afterward, some doctors allow almost unlimited weight gain, while others are more stringent. We offer you a new perspective on this issue and provide you with new data so that you can decide for yourself.

3. **Overcoming Postpartum Depression:** Many of you know first-hand how debilitating postpartum depression can be. You might not be aware that there seems to be a far more common, yet subtle, form of postpartum depression that can derail your weight loss efforts. Depression and weight loss do not go well together, especially if you were overweight before your pregnancy. The good news is that this is one mind game that you can win.

4. **Avoiding and Controlling Gestational Diabetes:** The diabetes of pregnancy, which affects 150,000 women in this country each year and millions worldwide, can derail not only your weight loss but your overall health, too. It is imperative that you talk to your doctor and find out whether you have any of the risk factors for gestational diabetes and, if so, how to protect yourself. This is a health issue fraught with misunderstanding by both the public and the medical community. Chapter Ten will clear everything up for you.

5. **Establishing the Mind-set of Working Women:** Researchers have been very perplexed by this factor. Women who return to a paying job lose more weight—and lose it faster—than those who remain at home. Why should this be? It's not simply due to working mothers' being out of the house, because women who work as volunteers or in any non-paying job out of the home do not fare as well. We need to explore the

mind-set of the women returning to work. In fact, the second weight loss trimester reveals a possible biochemical reason for this incredible phenomenon. When we look at this issue more closely, you will be able to glean valuable insights into a new factor of weight loss success, whether you work or not.

There, you have the five keys in hand. Each of them is incorporated in the *Hello, Baby! Good-bye, Baby Fat!* weight loss plan. You may think that factors such as the weight gain of pregnancy and gestational diabetes play important roles only during pregnancy. Not true! These two factors in particular can influence your weight after you deliver. Part III is devoted to these two pregnancy-related factors.

Even if you are about to deliver or have recently delivered, Part III will still give you valuable insight into both weight loss and your long-term health. This is especially true if you plan on getting pregnant again.

These factors of success may seem unrelated to each other. By the time you finish this book, however, you will understand that they are intertwined and work together to help cement your postpartum weight loss success.

Chapter Five

Are You the Weight Loss Type?

When you were inside your mother's womb, your first factor in postpartum weight loss success was already set. That's right, it was part of your parents' legacy to you: your genes. Not those Levi's jeans that you're aiming to get into, but your *genes!*

Is your family tall? Are they good athletes? Not all families are as smart as yours. Certain families are taller than others; some families have members that can run faster or jump higher, or have better vision or less incidence of heart disease or cancer. All of these attributes are felt to be hereditary. They are passed, more or less from one generation to the next, via genes. Even longevity is gene-related and runs in families. Weight gain and the potential for weight loss are no different. Like playing the violin or singing, some people are just genetically better at weight loss than others. Unfortunately, this talent is spread unevenly through the population. You probably know someone who tries every method of weight loss possible but still struggles daily without results. She tries everything from starving herself to the latest miracle fat-busting pill, all with negative results.

Then there is that next-door neighbor everyone seems to have. You know who I mean. She's the one who just had a baby and regained her figure in twelve minutes or less—or so it seems. She's probably the same neighbor who eats anything she wants and doesn't put on an ounce of weight. (I've never actually met this universal neighbor, and I don't know if anyone has. She could just be a part of a collective desire to believe that weight loss can be achieved effortlessly, or rather to place it entirely in the domain of American mythology, like Paul Bunyan and his ox, Babe.)

Just about all of your mental and physical traits follow rules that are made by your genes. These genetic rules also apply to the amount of weight that you gain during pregnancy and lose following delivery. The postpartum period will bring out the best of your weight loss potential, but this doesn't mean that if you weighed 250 pounds during your pregnancy you will automatically weigh 125 pounds afterward. Your goal should not be to look like that infamous next-door neighbor of yours. Your goal should be more personal and individualized. You should strive to lose as much weight during the postpartum as your genetic potential and your life's circumstances will allow.

Clichés abound throughout pregnancy and the postpartum. However, there is one cliché that, while steeped in the lore of the old wives' tale, still has definite scientific merit: "You tend to carry like Mommy, Grandma, and Aunt Sally." There is a strong correlation between the amount of weight *you* gain and how much your mom, your grandmother, and perhaps your maternal aunt gained. Since the weight gain of pregnancy and the amount of weight retained afterward are directly related, you can use this relationship to plot your own weight loss future. In an effort to determine exactly how family history contributes to a woman's weight loss outcome, I interviewed almost two thousand formerly pregnant women. I asked them questions about both their own and their relatives' weight gain in pregnancy and weight loss after delivery. It soon became apparent that there are three different patterns of weight loss in women. More important, we could predict postpartum weight loss outcomes of all three types by comparing how much weight the new mother gained and lost with the amounts gained and lost by her mother or grandmother.

I call the three types Type A, Type B, and Type C. Desirable-weight new moms, whom I call Type A moms, lose most of their weight during the first trimester of weight loss—that is, in the first few months, or sometimes weeks, after delivery.

Type B new moms are overweight. They tend to lose their weight by the end of the second weight loss trimester, or five to six months.

Type C new moms are obese. They are more apt to need more time to slim down postpartum. Obese new moms who breast-feed do best in the third weight loss trimester, or six months after delivery.

No matter what type you are, you still have the potential to lose enough weight to weigh less than you did *before* you were pregnant.

Let's see what type you are.

NEW MOMS, IDENTIFY YOURSELVES

Type A Moms

Our Type A new mom is of desirable weight and has thin wrists and ankles. We call her "small-boned." She has never been overweight, has no history of obesity in the family, and has no problem following her doctor's recommendation of limiting her pregnancy weight gain to 25 or 30 pounds. Her mother, who also has no history of being over-weight, was told to gain only 20 pounds when she was pregnant, which she did. Mom lost all her weight within three months of delivery, and has had no subsequent problem with obesity, diabetes, or hyperten-sion. Type A new moms may have a sister with a similar history.

If this scenario describes you, then you have some potent weight loss factors working in your favor. You are in the weight loss driver's seat. Your genetic background favors weight loss, and your mission, there-fore, is simple. Follow the suggestions in this book and learn about the three trimesters of weight loss so that you don't sabotage your body's natural ability to lose weight.

The major key to your success is to gain no more than 30 to 35 pounds during pregnancy. A fascinating thing about Type A's such as yourself is that you rarely lose much weight beyond your initial pre-pregnancy weight. This is easily understandable. You had little fat on your body to begin with, and little to lose in the end.

Being a Type A can have a negative side, though. Some Type A's may have a history of excessive exercise or eating disorders. These may lead to too-rapid weight loss, and studies show that new moms who lose weight too quickly are actually at risk of *gaining* weight by year's end! They are also at risk of not gaining enough weight during pregnancy, which can be dangerous to the fetus. Many teenagers fall into this cat-egory.

Type B Moms

While there are plenty of Type A's around, there are many more Type B's. Chances are you are one of them. Type B moms are borderline overweight before pregnancy. They may have been thin as children and put on some weight after puberty or in their late teens. Type B's have thick wrists and ankles, and we call them "large-boned." They usually have a normal amount of fat cells in their bodies and at conception usually weigh more than a Type A does at delivery.

The amount of weight Type B's put on during pregnancy varies greatly and can range from 25 to 75 pounds or even more! A look at the family history shows that diabetes and high blood pressure are present, and in fact one parent may recently have been put on blood-pressure medication. A Type B woman's mother may have developed a "touch" of diabetes during her pregnancy that was treated by diet changes only. If you are a Type B, your mother may have gained 45 pounds carrying you and perhaps the same amount or more carrying your brother or sister. At delivery, a Type B's mom may have weighed 185 pounds, and after breast-feeding for a few months, she probably lost most, but not all, of her pregnancy weight. Unfortunately, she now has developed a bit of a stomach and has been battling her weight ever since her second child was born.

If this scenario describes you and your family, you need to pay close attention to the program! You are not as genetically well endowed as a Type A, but you have a lot more going for you than you think. In fact, the women in this group have the greatest potential to lose enough weight to go below their pre-pregnancy weight! This is what happened to Debbie, whom you met in Chapter One, and it can happen to you.

But one thing is clear. If you are to keep weight off in the future, you cannot remain more than a few pounds or so above your pre-pregnancy weight. Your success will be based on how well you do in the second trimester of weight loss. The downside to being a Type B is the potential, especially when there is excessive weight gain during pregnancy, to be among the future obese of this country. To avoid this unsavory possibility, you need to do something about it now.

Type C Moms

Type C's are women who were obese, or 20 percent or more above ideal body weight, before pregnancy. Their bodies vary in shape from "apples" to "pears," depending upon where their body fat is concentrated. Prior to conception, they weigh what Type B's might weigh when pregnant. It is estimated that 10 to 15 percent of all women fall into this category, and the number is growing. Chances are that a Type C mom will have been obese since childhood and may be a high-risk pregnancy now. Many woman have menstrual and fertility problems, and may have taken fertility drugs that can make them even heavier. Type C new moms usually have an abnormally high number of fat cells, which helps perpetuate their obesity. Type C's also have strong family histories of obesity along with diabetes and high blood pressure. There is a good chance that a Type C's mom, aunt, or grandmother had gestational diabetes, and heart disease is prevalent on both sides of the family. High cholesterol may lurk in the family history as well.

Interestingly, Type C's tend to gain the least weight during pregnancy and lose the most weight after! This does not mean that you will automatically lose 60 to 70 pounds after delivery. It does mean that since these women historically have lost lots of weight in the postpartum period, your weight loss prognosis is good: The key to your success may be long-term lifestyle changes, including breast-feeding. Losing weight in the postpartum may be your only chance to attain a healthy lifetime weight!

Here are three charts that summarize the features of typical Type A, Type B, and Type C new moms.

TYPE A: DESIRABLE-WEIGHT NEW MOMS

Pre-Pregnancy Weight—desirable, normal weight

Body Type—thin wrists and ankles, "small-boned"

Pregnancy Weight Gain—30 pounds or less

Obstetrical History—two other children, gained less than 35 pounds each time

Weight Retained Following Last Delivery—half a pound

Family Obstetrical History—mother gained 19 pounds with each of two children, retained 1 pound

Family History of Diabetes or Obesity—no

Chance of Going Beyond Pre-Pregnancy Weight—slight

Weight Loss Prognosis—excellent overall

Comments—Breast-feeding plays no role in weight loss with these mothers. Some of these women have eating disorders such as bulimia and often have trouble gaining weight in pregnancy. Lacking a genetic predisposition to obesity, they are quick to shed excess fat.

TYPE B: OVERWEIGHT NEW MOMS

Pre-Pregnancy Weight—overweight
Body Type—thick wrists and ankles, "large-boned"
Pregnancy Weight Gain—varies widely between 25 and 75 pounds, or more
Obstetrical History—one child, gained 44 pounds
Weight Retained Following Last Delivery—9 pounds after one year
Family Obstetrical History—sister developed gestational diabetes, mother retained 12 pounds with each of two children and is now obese
Family History of Diabetes or Obesity—yes
Chance of Going Beyond Pre-Pregnancy Weight—yes
Weight Loss Prognosis—excellent
Comments—These moms should limit the amount of weight that they gain in pregnancy. They can develop gestational diabetes. They have a normal number of fat cells, which makes their weight loss easier than it is for Type C's.

TYPE C: OBESE NEW MOMS

Pre-Pregnancy Weight—obese
Body Type—obese, with large waist/hip ratio; can be "apples" or "pears"
Pregnancy Weight Gain—often 20 pounds or less, but the range can be large, as with Type B's
Obstetrical History—first pregnancy, has used fertility drugs
Weight Retained Following Last Delivery—not applicable
Family Obstetrical History—mother had gestational diabetes with three different children, all born large; also had high blood pressure when pregnant
Family History of Diabetes or Obesity—strong family history of adult-onset diabetes and obesity on both sides of the family

continued

Chance of Going Beyond Pre-Pregnancy Weight—possible

Comments—These new moms usually gain the least weight of any group, but they are more apt to have complications in childbirth because they may bear large babies. Breast-feeding may play a large weight loss role for these women. They often take fertility drugs to resolve problems caused by menstrual difficulties at a young age. They have an abnormal number of fat cells in their bodies. These fat cells never go away, which explains why Type C's often do not reach their goal weight.

Three different types of new moms, with three different weight loss histories and weight loss prognoses. Before you read the next part of this book, in which we return often to discussions of these types, be sure you know which type of new mom you are.

To find out how you figure into this classification, try to obtain your family's obstetrical history. Ask your parents, your sisters, your aunts, and your grandparents. Look for family photos; they are the source for determining how much a relative weighed when pregnant, since it is common for people to understate their real weight. Finding photos may be difficult because many cultures look upon taking pictures of pregnant women as casting a spell or an "evil eye." Also, many women feel uncomfortable about being photographed while pregnant. How many pictures do you have of yourself while pregnant? Still, find out whatever you can. Your postpartum weight loss success can be greatly enhanced the more you know.

I hope that this new understanding of your genetic postpartum weight loss potential has also reinforced the fact that there is no need to compare yourself to others because each one of you is unique, special.

Guidance for your first trimester of weight loss is now only a page or two away. No matter what your potential for postpartum weight loss is, with proper guidance and attitude you will learn how to outsmart your genes and fit into your new jeans!

Part II

The Three
Postpartum
Trimesters
of Weight Loss

Chapter Six

Birth to Three Months Postpartum: The First Trimester of Weight Loss

Congratulations! You just became a new mom, and your postpartum weight loss adventure has begun. We call the first three months following delivery a new mom's first trimester of weight loss. Over the next ninety days you are going to lose a lot of weight, but at this moment, you probably feel like you just ran the New York City Marathon!

Your heart is racing; sweat is pouring. Muscles that you didn't even know you had are sore, and will be for days. Even your lungs hurt from breathing so hard. You feel a fatigue like at no other time in your life, and all you want is a chance to sleep—for about three weeks!

For the past few hours strangers have been cheering you on, calling out, "Come on, you can do it," or, "Push! Push!" or, "Just a bit more—you're almost at the finish line." Finally, after your baby is born, someone offers you a small cup of water for your parched lips.

It does sound like a marathon, but what you have just been through is labor! No more appropriate word has ever described a human activity. Labor is even tougher than running a marathon. Well, it's over and you did it! After what you have been through, weight loss will be *easy*.

I hope that you and your baby are healthy and doing well. Those of you who required a cesarean section have had your own tribulations, and I hope that you, too, are resting and in little pain.

For the past 270 days, many of your bodily functions—including your weight—were controlled in part by the placenta, which has now left your body. In an instant, and without your feeling a thing, your body has switched gears, transformed from a nine-month weight gain machine into a prime-time weight loss dynamo.

Such a profound change in such a short time is rarely seen in nature. Another example is that of hibernating bears, who gain lots of fat for their winter's sleep. They too are in a weight gain mode for months. With the arrival of spring, bears suddenly awake, emerge into the fresh air, and quickly lose any remaining excess weight.

It's understandable that few women are concerned with weight loss immediately after childbirth, but events are rapidly unfolding in your body that you should know about. They will give you the weight loss head start that you need in order to weigh less than you did before you were pregnant.

Speaking of head starts, if you plan to breast-feed, you should begin within an hour of birth. This idea is based on the new breast-feeding guidelines issued in late 1997 by the American Academy of Pediatrics. They are radically different from previous recommendations, and your doctor or nurse should review them with you. We detail breast-feeding and weight loss issues, including the new recommendations, in Chapter Eight.

Many of you are under the impression that your weight loss efforts should not begin until six weeks after delivery. That's because under normal circumstances, your first follow-up visit with your doctor is set at six weeks postpartum, which is the average point in time at which a non-breast-feeding woman's uterus has contracted, or shrunk to its normal size (about the size and shape of a pear). This is a major signpost of your physical recuperation, and your doctor may use it to gauge your recovery.

I strongly disagree with the idea of waiting six weeks before beginning your weight loss efforts. As we've noted, as soon as you deliver the placenta, tremendous changes begin taking place inside you. Your body is all set to start losing weight, and you can do it! I know that you are tired and energy is at a premium, but no one is asking you to jump out of bed and rush to a gym. You don't have to! I told you this would be a lot easier than that!

After your short stay in the unreal world of the hospital, you return to the real world of your home. Sooner or later, we both know that your weight will become a concern, so I propose a compromise. Let your physical condition dictate when you begin your weight loss efforts.

Don't get bogged down by some artificial time barrier, such as the six-week mark. Certainly those of you who had complications with your delivery (such as a cesarean section) will need more time to heal, but for the majority of you new moms there is no reason to wait. Let's get going!

Whatever you do, don't feel guilty or lazy because you can't muster the energy of that trim, sun-tanned fitness guru featured in the post-partum exercise video you bought. There is absolutely no need for you to exercise now if you don't want to. You already know that exercise is not the key to postpartum weight loss, anyway.

Do it at your own pace and in your own style. Remember, you already have lost lots of weight. Like all new moms, you are already the greatest weight loss champion of all time! Just look at your tally in the first 24 hours after delivery.

YOUR WEIGHT LOSS: THE FIRST 24 HOURS

The immediate steps your body takes in an effort to restore itself are nothing short of astounding. Just think of your baby sliding down your birth canal to daylight, stretching your ligaments, muscles, bladder, and other tissues. Your leg and belly veins are engorged. Your liver, kidneys, heart, and lungs have also undergone changes in their internal architecture over the past nine months. All must return to "the way they were," so your body wastes no time putting these body parts back in the right places. This process of self-repair is one of the miracles of life and comes from an unknown signal deep in your body. Self-repair begins at birth, goes on 24 hours a day, and can last up to a year. Weight loss, which makes up a big part of this self-renewal project, also begins right at birth. Here is a breakdown of the weight loss you should experience on your first day as new mother. Some of you will lose more weight, some less, but this is what most of you can expect:

WEIGHT LOSS ALL IN ONE DAY

GOOD-BYE BABY WEIGHT: The average American woman gains just over 30 pounds and delivers a baby that weighs about seven and a half pounds. ....7.5 pounds

GOOD-BYE WEIGHTY PLACENTA: The placenta which followed your baby into this world weighed about one and a half pounds. ....1.5 pounds

GOOD-BYE WATER: During delivery you may have noticed that your baby and the placenta were covered in fluid. This is the amniotic fluid that surrounds your baby in the uterus, and it acts as a shock absorber. When you say, "My water broke," you are talking about this amniotic fluid. It weighs a total of about two pounds. ....2 pounds

Total Weight Loss the First Day ....11 pounds

---

So far, from just delivery alone, you are, on average, 11 pounds lighter, all in one day! When have you done that before? Before you pat yourself on the back, though, let's take a closer look at what's ahead.

Suppose you gained 30 pounds during your pregnancy. Subtract the 11 pounds that you lose at delivery, and you are left with 19 pounds. Are these 19 pounds of fat? No! Thank goodness, no! In fact, only half of this weight, or about 10 pounds, is fat. Much of the rest is made up of extra tissue that you accumulated over the past nine months. That means you still have another round of weight loss coming your way.

During the next few weeks, much of your remaining weight will be shed automatically, except for the increased breast weight of breast-feeding moms. As your body continues its internal repair job, you once again lose weight as a by-product. Below is a list of some of the weight changes that your body will undergo during round two of your immediate postpartum weight loss. (Remember, all of these weights are averages; the amount that you lose could be more or less than these figures.)

YOUR WEIGHT LOSS: THE FIRST FEW WEEKS

YOU WILL LOSE THE EXTRA BLOOD THAT YOU FORMED: The amount of blood in your body increased to provide the extra nutrients that your developing baby needed. A good part of this increased blood volume was due to your not having a monthly period during pregnancy. Say good-bye to this new blood, which weighs a total of about 3 pounds. ....3 pounds

YOUR ENLARGED UTERUS WILL SHRINK: The change in the size and shape of your uterus is probably the most profound postpartum body change you will experience, besides, of course, the delivery of the baby and placenta. During pregnancy, your uterus swelled up to about 2½ pounds; within a few weeks it will weigh a few ounces. Women who breast-feed will have a quicker shrinkage of their uterus. ....3 pounds

YOUR ENLARGED BREASTS WILL RETURN TO NORMAL: Whether you breast-feed or not, your breasts have enlarged in anticipation of breast-feeding. They now each weigh 1 pound extra, for a total of 2 pounds. They will revert to their former size unless, of course, you breast-feed..2 pounds

THE EXTRA FLUID IN YOUR BODY DISAPPEARS: For the last nine months your body needed to hold on to more water than usual. This extra fluid helped support all of the new tissues discussed above, and weighed approximately 3 pounds (more in women who had edema, or fluid buildup, during pregnancy). Sometimes women develop a permanent problem with extra fluid after delivery, but for most of you this extra fluid is urinated out of your body for good.   ....3 pounds

TOTAL AUTOMATIC WEIGHT LOSS, FIRST FEW WEEKS: ....11 pounds
Add up all this silent weight loss, and after a few weeks you are down another 11 pounds, bringing your total weight loss to about 22 pounds! Remember you still haven't done anything to promote weight loss—it has all just happened according to nature's plan.

After your body completes the second round of weight loss, any excess weight that remains is fat.

If you are a Type A, desirable-weight new mom, and you gained the average 30 pounds during your pregnancy, you are left with only 8 pounds of fat to lose in order to be back to where you were before you were pregnant. Lose just one pound more, and you will join the ranks of the 400,000 women who now weigh *less* than before!

Is 8 pounds a lot of weight to lose? Of course not, especially with that special postpartum body of yours leading the way!

But those of you who have gained lots of weight during pregnancy are looking at a different picture. The more weight you gained above what you and your baby needed for normal growth and development, the greater the percentage of your excess body weight that is fat. Some women gain so much excess weight that 60 percent of their total pregnancy weight is made up of fat! Watch what happens with larger weight gains.

Suppose you gain 50 pounds during your pregnancy and deliver a 10-pound baby. Like all postpartum women, over the next few weeks you will automatically shed the tissues we discussed above, also known as the products of conception, which weigh about 15 pounds. This will leave you weighing an extra 25 pounds. Instead of 8 pounds of excess weight, you are left with 25 pounds to lose. These 25 pounds are fat. As we all know, it's a lot easier to lose 8 pounds than 25!

If this sounds like you, you are still in luck because the postpartum holds out the promise of weight loss for everyone, no matter what she weighs.

HOME AT LAST

After a few days, depending on your and your baby's medical conditions (and the type of insurance you have!), you arrive home. Isn't there something special about carrying your baby all bundled up, safe and secure, through your front door for the first time?

My first piece of advice is, don't jump on the scale just yet. If you are the type of person who weighs herself every ten minutes and you do go ahead and get on that scale, don't be surprised if you don't see weight loss over the next few days, especially if you delivered via cesarean section. Some new moms may actually gain a pound or two during the first few days after delivery. British scientists examined this issue over twenty-five years ago and concluded that this slight weight gain is due to water retention (*edema*). More important, they found that this water weight does not interfere with your weight loss.

At about this time, most new moms like you begin to lose their excess fat. That's because your body is entering the weight loss mode that we have been talking about. It's time for you to begin—

EATING FOR ONE AGAIN!

At around the fifth postpartum day, three sudden changes take place inside you. Each is better than the next, and together they pack a hefty weight loss punch. They are:

- Your appetite is suppressed.
- Your metabolism goes up.
- Your ability to hold on to fat goes down.

Once baby and placenta have left your body, the powerful biological drive that governed pregnancy and urged you to eat officially ends. Instead of having to eat for two, now you barely have to eat for one. That's because your hormones tell your "old" pregnancy appetite to take a hike and, in a flash, your appetite is suppressed. There is no need for willpower, starvation, or self-denial, because your body does a much better job suppressing your appetite naturally. Hormones that promote hunger, such as estrogen and progesterone, are no longer ordering you to eat all those mass quantities of pickles and ice cream, as they did when you were pregnant. (This situation is different for those of you who breast-feed, as you shall see in Chapter Eight.) This sudden anti-food hormonal swing explains why you rarely hear of new moms being ravenous unless they have postpartum depression. In fact, most non-breast-feeding new moms whom I interviewed could barely recall what they ate, let alone their attitude about food, following delivery. That's because the sudden appetite suppression they experienced made them care less about food. It also allowed them to feel fuller on less food, and eat less, period.

How long does this natural appetite suppression last? Your "old" appetite will not return for months because your hormones have temporarily lost interest in monitoring your food intake. They have far more feminine things to take care of, like restoring your regular menstrual cycle to enable you to reproduce again (if you want to!).

Remember what we said about hormones: Unlike people or even angels, they can do two things at once. Your sex hormones, estrogen and progesterone, not only promote weight gain but also orchestrate your menstrual cycle. Following delivery, these sex hormones concentrate solely on your period. They have to, because for the past nine months your pregnancy has caused you to skip your period, a condition known as *amenorrhea*.

Eventually your period will return, if you have regular cycles. It might take two months or longer (much longer if you breast-feed) but it's going to happen either in this first trimester of weight loss or by the middle of the second.

In the meantime, besides controlling appetite suppression, your hormones are encouraging further weight loss by increasing your metabolism and making life miserable for fat. This kind of intense weight loss–favoring hormonal activity only occurs once in your life, in the first trimester of weight loss. These are precisely the biochemical changes that allow you to weigh *less* than before your pregnancy.

THE WEIGHT LOSS BATTLE OF THE SEXES!

Women often lament that the weight loss cards are stacked against them. In particular, two things seem totally unfair. First, men lose weight a lot more easily than women do and second, a woman's metabolism slows with age, making weight loss more difficult.

If you have always believed that this inequality exists, you were absolutely right! There *is* a gender weight loss gap! Women do not fare as well as men in the weight loss arena because a woman's internal chemistry usually promotes weight gain and makes shedding body fat more difficult. In addition, there is a metabolic age gap. After age 22, your metabolism slows, and continues to do so as you age.

A turnabout now is fair play. The postpartum period is the great gender-bender and metabolic equalizer. That's because your hormones are practically fighting each other to help you lose weight. Besides your diminished appetite and elevated metabolism, your delivery has created a temporary hormonal imbalance that makes it tough for you to accumulate new fat. Here is a closer look at the parade of hormone changes taking place inside of you.

Estrogen and progesterone, the two chief female hormones, have plummeted because they were made by the now-gone and all-but-forgotten placenta. These two hormones may separate the women from the boys, but they also foster female weight gain. Estrogen increases your appetite while progesterone makes it easy for your body to deposit fat all over your body. With these two fatmongers lying low for a few months, you are not only less hungry but your body will find it more difficult than ever to widen your hips, thighs, and buttocks.

Leptin is a recently discovered "fat-melting" hormone that also raises your metabolism. The latest research suggests that leptin plays an important role in the regulation of your body weight and in your ability to reproduce. Leptin reaches a high level in your blood during pregnancy and then falls rapidly at delivery. As you will see in Chapter Seven, leptin plays an important role in determining how much fat you ultimately will retain. Having leptin on your side, for once, allows you to do what Debbie in Chapter One and 400,000 new moms do each year: Overcome your set point!

Insulin is the hormone that controls the level of sugar in your blood. Insulin also plays a vital role in weight control. All pregnant women, especially overweight new moms, make more insulin than usual. High levels of insulin in your blood not only make you hungrier but increase your body's ability to paste on fat. That's because insulin likes to push fat into fat cells. The more insulin you have, the more fat can be shoved in and stored in your fat cells. Now, following delivery, your insulin level falls and, with it, your appetite and your ability to deposit fat.

Fat lipase is an enzyme that, like insulin, is made in the pancreas. It is responsible for all phases of fat metabolism, from the initial absorption of fat from your food right up to the actual placing of fat in the fat cells of your thighs, your hips, and elsewhere. In this latter capacity, fat lipase can be thought of as performing insulin's "dirty work," because it works together with insulin to fill your fat cells with fat. During pregnancy, fat lipase becomes overly active. After delivery, fat lipase lies dormant for a while, making it difficult for your body to accumulate fat.

And there is more. . . .

Endorphins are substances in the brain that influence both what goes into your mouth and your mood. Most of you know endorphins as the brain chemical responsible for the so-called "runner's high." This is the near-orgasmic feeling that athletes experience after sustained hard physical activity. It is believed that this emotional "rush" is caused by the hypothalamus gland in your brain secreting more and more endorphins into your blood. Endorphins are also released by your brain when you are under stress and during sex (try making vigorous love when you are stressed.) Unfortunately, while endorphins may make you feel better, they also make you eat more. This helps explain why you tend to chow down when stressed, after a hard game of tennis, or after great sex! However, in the immediate postpartum period endorphin levels fall, making you less likely to binge in times of stress. This is perfect timing because the postpartum, as you know, is just full of stress.

CALORIES TAKE A HOLIDAY

Everything is going your way weight loss–wise. It will take months for your hormones, enzymes, and metabolism to revert to pre-pregnancy levels. While this weight loss–favoring hormonal imbalance is in charge, you becomes very sensitive to slight decreases in your food intake and slight increases in your activity level. Even calories become your friend for once!

It seems as if the whole calorie theory takes a holiday during pregnancy and in the postpartum. We all know about calories, the energy content of food. We count them, we measure them, we hate them! We also know that it is the increased calories that you take in from your food that account for your baby's (and your) growth and development during pregnancy, and for any excess weight, as well.

During the last six months of your pregnancy, you consumed on average an extra 300 to 500 calories a day. This small daily increase doesn't seem like much, but over six months it adds up to 80,000 extra calories. That's a lot of calories! To gain one pound, you need to ingest 3200 calories above what you normally eat. If you divide 80,000 calories by 3200 calories you can account for the average American 30-pound pregnancy weight gain—or can you?

Scientists have long been puzzled by the lack of correlation between the number of calories eaten during pregnancy and the amount of weight gained. Pregnant women, it seems, are able to gain weight out of proportion to the amount of food that they eat. In other words, they gain a lot of weight despite eating small quantities of food. Somehow the body of a pregnant woman becomes super-efficient at holding on to fat, especially in the "problem areas" of the thighs, hips, and buttocks. No one has yet figured out why this is so.

After your baby is born, this trend reverses itself. Now, for reasons that we once again do not fully understand, your body makes it hard for fat to accumulate on your thighs, hips, and buttocks. Did you ever think of your body as a fat fighter? Well, it is! Now see what your body can do to help your metabolism when it wants to.

HOME LIPOSUCTION 101

With each passing day of your pregnancy, you became heavier and less active. With a protruding belly tugging on your spinal column, causing your back to ache fiercely, and with your swollen feet pulsating with pain, you had little inclination to move. Eventually you slowed to a crawl. One study has compared the activity level of a late-term mother to that of a lazy high school "couch potato!" Honest! I couldn't make that one up!

Now, everyone knows that when you exercise you raise your metabolism, and when you are sedentary you lower it, right? Wrong! Pregnant women are different! Despite a lower activity level, the metabolic rate of a pregnant woman goes *up*, not down. In fact the heavier you are, the *higher* your metabolism goes! And your metabolism rate will remain high for the first few months after delivery. It is estimated that your metabolism rises an average of about 13 percent above normal. That's a lot! It is a true gift of nature that you will never receive again. Breast-feeding women, by the way, have the highest and most sustained rates of metabolism.

Remember the last part of your pregnancy—when you were so tired that your head seemed glued to the pillow? After delivery, your normal increase in activity inside and outside your home keeps your metabolism high naturally. No need to do sit-ups or trek to a gym, and no, you don't have to remove the clothes you leave drying on that exercise machine in your bedroom, either. Your body burns fat quite well without their help, thank you.

Think of your metabolism as a burning fire, a fire that is now raging. To continue burning so brightly, a constant supply of fuel is needed. The fuel, of course, is your food. Your higher metabolism needs more fuel now, just as it did when you were pregnant. However, after delivery your appetite is decreased, not increased as it was during the past nine months. You have created a mismatch between your metabolism, which is high, and your food intake, which is low. Should you eat the same amount of food now that you did before you were pregnant, it will not be enough to keep up with your new metabolism. Sensing this, your body demands an immediate backup fuel source to maintain your higher metabolic rate.

Help arrives quickly from the fat on your hips, thighs, and buttocks. Desperately needing a new energy source, your body attacks and breaks down any extra stored fat that you have and then burns it as fuel. This process is known as *fat catabolism*. Powerful hormones and enzymes can turn mounds of fat into small fat droplets, which circulate in your system. Eventually these tiny pieces of fat get taken up and are burned by your muscles. Is this "home liposuction" or what?

You don't need an advanced degree in physiology to realize that any time your body is breaking up your fat, you are going to lose weight. Without any formal exercise your body behaves as if it's on a 24-hour treadmill.

The best part is that your body does not care when you first put the extra fat on your body. Fat that you had on your body *before* you were pregnant gets consumed with as much ease as fat that you put on *with* your pregnancy. Now you understand why so many women use the word "melt" when describing their weight loss after delivery.

Your journey to weighing less begins with some simple math. Following delivery your body is still geared up for your old pregnancy weight and the additional 300 to 500 calories per day that you took in. Now, with a diminished appetite, an elevated metabolism, and with your body burning fat and unable to accumulate new fat easily, you are in a total weight loss mode. By modifying your old pre-pregnancy eating habits (even if they weren't so great) with the *Hello, Baby! Good-bye, Baby Fat!* eating and lifestyle plan, you can begin to subtract calories! It's a beautiful thing!

Depending upon your initial weight and your activity level, a typical Type A new mom with 10 pounds or so to lose can be finished with the program in as little as three to four weeks. This means that for most Type A new moms, and for some Type B's, this first weight loss trimester may also be their last! Again, nursing moms have a different pattern of weight loss, as you shall see in Chapter Eight.

Those of you who are extremely overweight or obese will need more time than just a few weeks. Your weight loss efforts will need to continue into the next two trimesters of weight loss. The good news is, however, that the heavier you are, the more weight you lose over time. It is not unusual to find overweight and obese new moms losing 30 pounds or more during the first trimester of weight loss!

Some obese women, like 34-year-old Mary C.—"hard luck" weight-loser in the past—shed more than 5 pounds a week during the first weight loss trimester. Eventually Mary lost 95 pounds, going from a pregnancy weight of 220 down to 125 pounds. She is now a spokesperson for a national weight loss chain and does the lecture circuit. You may have seen her on T.V. hawking the latest diet aid. Her pregnancy was the catalyst behind her success, just as yours will be.

Mary's marvelous outcome illustrates the wonderful weight loss potential inside you as a result of giving birth.

In a perfect world, every new mom should be able to accomplish what Mary did. You will be amazed to discover, as I was, that there are two major stumbling blocks that new moms face that can stop them from reaching their true weight loss potential. Both problems involve self-sabotage. In one instance, you knowingly sabotage your body. In the second instance, your *body* unknowingly sabotages you! But both of these problems are easily correctable.

NO STARVING ARTISTS ALLOWED

Since your body does not come with an owner's manual, it is not unusual for a person to try to fix things that aren't broken. The time after delivery is not the time to tinker. Far too many new moms sabotage their own weight loss efforts by playing too much of the old dieting and starvation game.

The biggest mistake a new mom can make now is to go on a low calorie or starvation diet. I consider a low calorie diet one that contains fewer than 1100 calories per day for an average-sized woman. Some women I know have even tried the so-called "very low calorie diets" (VLCDs) that consist of consuming fewer than 800 calories per day.

Your body is trying to restore itself, and it needs proper nutrition to do so. Consider this: Besides requiring extra vitamins such as B_6 and folic acid, and minerals such as calcium and zinc, after nine months of excess food intake, your body is searching for nutritional balance. You need to eat in a way that will not only amplify your body's process of self-repair (which includes weight loss) but that will also restore the body's balance of protein, fat, and carbohydrates. Starving yourself or trying a fad high-protein or high-fat diet now will do nothing for you but totally mess up the works. Obviously, we are assuming that you are not breast-feeding. Breast-feeding new moms should never drastically cut their food intake.

Also, severe dieting now will counter the three postpartum weight loss hormonal changes that we outlined above. Go on a fad diet when your body is giving you a free weight loss ride and say "so long" to your diminished appetite and decreased ability to deposit fat. Instead, say "hello" to a newly increased appetite and ability to pack on the fat. Worse still, severe dieting does the one thing that will terminate your weight loss. It lowers your metabolism.

A study conducted at UCLA showed that your metabolic rate is slowed by up to 40 percent when fewer than 1000 calories are consumed per day! That's like cutting your metabolism in half! Not only are you not going to get thinner, you are going to gain weight, and quickly too! In fact, a 40 percent decrease in the metabolism of an overweight woman can translate into a 30-pound weight gain over the course of a year! Why on earth would you want to lower your metabolism?

Don't think that you will buck the odds, either. Sure, going on a fad diet will let you lose a few pounds now, but watch how things change. Many new moms who lose weight too quickly will actually gain weight after a few months, and this weight gain becomes permanent.

And there is yet another reason why new moms should not be stingy with their food. All new moms experience fatigue, sleep disturbances, and mood swings after giving birth. What you eat in the postpartum period will go a long way toward increasing your energy level and normalizing your mood and sleeping patterns.

Don't sabotage the natural weight loss mode that you are in. Eat your way to success! Your body knows exactly what it's doing, and now *you* know exactly what your body is doing. During this all-important first weight loss trimester, the *Hello, Baby! Good-bye, Baby Fat!* eating and lifestyle plan gives your body exactly what it needs to allow you to weigh less than you did before you were pregnant.

Certainly, many new moms unwittingly sabotage their own efforts by the way that they eat, but to really change the way you look on the outside, you must come to grips with something that eats away at you, and sabotages your success—from the inside!

EMOTIONAL WEIGHT LOSS

As a new mom, you are thrown a curveball that plays with both your mind and your weight loss. You see, all the weight loss–promoting changes we have described so far can be negated by one body chemical that may not be acting in your favor. This body substance not only interferes with your weight loss but it can also make you sleep poorly, and feel depressed, fatigued, and unsexy. This chemical is present in your body in such small quantities that it is measured in billionths of a pound, yet it's so strong that I have seen it destroy the weight loss efforts of new moms weighing 115 or 215 pounds. What is it? This elusive biochemical culprit is none other than *serotonin*.

Serotonin is an important brain hormone, or *neurotransmitter*. At its normal level, serotonin will put you in a good mood and allow you to feel full on less food. It is nature's own appetite suppressor. Serotonin will also pique your interest in sex and help you sleep better. Mmmm, this sounds like fun stuff.

Think of serotonin as the metabolic glue that binds your mind to your body and keeps you level-headed, happy, sexy, and less preoccupied with food. You need to strengthen this connection because after delivery, serotonin levels fall, as do the levels of many other hormones and neurotransmitters. A fall in serotonin will unglue your mind/body connection, leaving you depressed, fatigued, irritable, unable to sleep, and unable to lose weight. In short, it can put a damper on your entire postpartum experience.

It is time to unmask this postpartum fall in serotonin for what it really is: one of the chief forces behind postpartum depression!

THE BABY BLUES

Watch out! After delivery, a mind-boggling foe can catch you by surprise. It's none other than postpartum depression, postpartum weight loss's Public Enemy Number One.

New moms often ride a wild roller coaster of emotions after delivery. At first you can be on a true "high," flooded with positive and warm feelings. A new mother's initial encounter and subsequent bonding with a newborn are such powerful and sublime events that women I have interviewed years later become choked with emotion when they are asked to describe their experiences.

Rina K., a 34-year-old travel agent, couldn't stop laughing when her son was born because she was so happy. Later she found herself crying because she didn't want the doctors or her husband to think she was crazy. It seems that crying feels more "appropriate" than laughing in the birthing room!

Another first-time mother, Barbara R., a 40-year-old office manager, told me that even though her birthing room had all the ambience of a newsstand at New York's Grand Central Station, she didn't want to leave the room after her daughter was born. It remains her favorite spot: Even today, twenty years later, she sometimes visits that room, and the decor hasn't changed!

But the postpartum emotional roller coaster comes down, too. You may feel lost and confused, out of control, racked with guilt or anxiety. Harvey Block, Ph.D., a psychologist in Bergen County, New Jersey, believes that the sudden transition from nine months of pregnancy to instant motherhood is too abrupt for many women, who now must trade the certainty of their old lives for the uncertainty of their new lives.

This explains why so many women use the word "bewildered" when describing the immediate postpartum. A woman's psyche can be burdened with questions such as, "Am I going to be a good mother?" or, "Should I return to work?" or, "Is my baby going to be healthy?" Many women also express great concern about their changed bodies and even their changed sex lives!

Birth can cause issues to surface that have been dormant and repressed for years, issues concerning the type of parents you had, for instance. Did you grow up in a loving family? What are your true feelings about your father and mother? Did you suffer any form of abuse? What is the real nature of your relationship with the father of your child? These questions can have happy or unhappy answers, and the period after birth often makes you confront them one by one.

Not helping matters much is that during this delicate time, during which you're likely to be sleep-deprived, some of your brain chemicals play tricks on you. Hormones that are responsible for your happy disposition under normal circumstances can now betray you by being nowhere to be found. These include not only serotonin, as we have discussed, but also endorphins and your sex hormones estrogen and progesterone. Their temporary hiatus, especially that of estrogen, can increase the scope and intensity of the negative vibes you feel, bringing you down, making you feel anxious, unable to sleep, weepy, or otherwise unable to enjoy the new mother experience as you should. If this is happening to you, you have entered the "baby blues" zone.

Consider the baby blues a touch of depression. About eight out of every ten women who deliver experience the baby blues. That's over three million women a year! The baby blues can begin at birth, or they can appear anytime in the first few weeks following delivery. E.M., an occupational therapist from California, described her baby blues as feeling trapped in a chase scene from her worst nightmare. She experienced crying spells, insomnia, drenching sweats, and constant lip-biting. After two weeks, E.M. recovered spontaneously. In fact, conventional wisdom claims that the baby blues depart on their own after a few days. Don't count on it! As you shall see, they often persist for months and can snowball into full-blown postpartum depression.

Our immediate concern with the baby blues, postpartum depression, and weight loss is well founded. Depression can block almost any attempt at weight loss.

Certain women are prone to the baby blues and postpartum depression. Women at risk include those with a history of depression and women who were sexually abused as children or adults. Below is a chart of postpartum depression risk factors for new moms. Keep in mind that any new mom, with or without any or all of these risk factors, can still get the baby blues and postpartum depression. The common denominator among all the risk factors is the "S" word: stress.

WOMEN AT RISK FOR POSTPARTUM DEPRESSION

Women at risk for the baby blues and postpartum depression
   include:
   • women with a personal history of depression
   • women who were sexually abused as children or adults
   • women with marital or financial problems
   • women who bore babies with medical problems
   • women who experienced multiple births
   • women who are single moms
   • women who experienced traumatic births

Even if you don't have any of these risk factors, and if you are for-
tunate enough not to suffer from postpartum depression, you are not
out of the woods just yet.

THE BABY BLAHS

Each year, between 500,000 and 800,000 new moms discover that
their baby blues develop into the more severe condition known as *postpartum depression*. Even mild cases of postpartum depression can
derail your weight loss because the link between depression and body
weight change is a strong one. Some Type A (desirable-weight) new
moms actually lose weight when depressed because they lose interest
in food. New moms who are overweight or obese often gain weight
when they are depressed because depression triggers their eating.
There is also a problem with time. Women consumed with depressed
thoughts show little inclination for weight loss. Time passes by, and
before you know it, the six-month weight loss barrier is reached and all
of your body's innate weight loss capabilities shut down. This is like
missing the "weight loss boat," and this is what helped derail Beth's
weight loss efforts detailed in Chapter One. Don't let it derail yours!

Since your hormones are the prime manipulators of your emotions,
postpartum depression can be thought of as a hormonal imbalance.
Postpartum depression, however, is not entirely biologically based.
Incredibly, it can also affect mothers who adopt! You would think that

since adoptive mothers do not experience the same internal biochemical changes that biological mothers do that they wouldn't experience postpartum depression. But they do!

Postpartum depression has also been observed in *men!* Both biological fathers and even adoptive fathers can be affected.

Don't minimize postpartum depression. Affected women should not be thought of as just being a bit "weepy." Postpartum depression is real and it is a universal phenomenon seen in all cultures, from industrialized Europe and Asia to the hunting and gathering peoples of the Amazon basin. If you have (or had) postpartum depression, then you know how far-reaching and debilitating its effects can be. Besides making weight loss tough or nearly impossible, there are quality of life issues to be considered as well.

Depressed new moms not only feel sad and tired and have low self-esteem but also have trouble concentrating and sleeping. Typically they lose interest in sex and anything pleasurable—including being mothers! Postpartum depression can be a harbinger of things to come. Many sufferers are destined to develop a severe depression sometime in the future.

Unfortunately, an even more sinister side to postpartum depression has come to light recently. Postpartum depression can have a profound effect on both a newborn and it's siblings, and this effect can last for a lifetime! Recent research focusing on the later development of children who had mothers with postpartum depression found that these children had negative impressions of their mothers, had an increased incidence of learning disabilities, and were more temperamental. Postpartum depression even negatively influences the way that these children will parent their own offspring. Amazingly, these observations all point out that the negative effects of postpartum depression are passed on not only to the second generation but can create problems for the third generation as well!

The spectrum of postpartum depression is a broad one. It ranges from the mildest case of the baby blues to the rare *postpartum psychosis,* an extremely dangerous situation in which a new mom loses touch with reality and may entertain suicidal thoughts about herself and homicidal feelings toward her child. Women suffering from postpartum psychosis need to be hospitalized immediately for their own and their babies' safety!

Nestled between the millions of annual cases of the baby blues and the hundreds of thousands of diagnosed cases of postpartum depression lie far more common and subtle cases of mental change that can dampen your weight loss efforts. I call this form of postpartum funk (which affects nearly *all* women who have recently delivered) the "baby blahs." Four symptoms make up the baby blahs. They are:

- Lack of energy
- Inability to sleep
- Mood swings
- Binge carbohydrate cravings (rare)

You may experience one or all of these symptoms. How many new mothers wish they could sleep better, or have more energy? How many of you have mood swings? Probably all of you! Binge carbohydrate cravings are not seen that often, thank goodness, and seem to affect only women with a history of depression. But in general these four symptoms are so common that they may even be considered a normal part of the postpartum experience. Why? Because the four symptoms of the baby blahs are most likely caused by the same drop in serotonin (and some of your sex hormones) that occurs in *all* women who have just delivered! These are the same hormonal changes that account for the major symptoms of postpartum depression, yet why certain women come down with the more severe type of depression, while others are just affected by the baby blahs, is unknown.

If the four symptoms of the baby blahs reminded you of premenstrual syndrome, or PMS, good for you! That's because after delivery your body is essentially awaiting the onset of your next menstrual period, just as it does during the premenstrual phase of your cycle. The underlying biochemistry is about the same too, with levels of serotonin falling, along with changes in estrogen and progesterone levels. As a result, many new moms now experience the mood swings, sleep problems, binge carbohydrate cravings, and fatigue that characterize PMS. Some new moms in the first few weeks after delivery describe themselves as feeling as if things are just a little "off," and as if no one understands what they are going through. While others glow over every move their new baby makes, these women sometimes just don't get the same enjoyment that others seem to. Many women have told me that they often don't want to leave the house during this time. Others have told me that tremendous sexual conflicts have arisen between them and their significant others.

A self-defeating attitude often predominates during the baby blahs: an attitude that thwarts the starting of any new projects, like weight loss. You need help. While your body is revved up to lose weight, your mind isn't! Who can you turn to?

I GET BY WITH A LITTLE HELP FROM . . .

If you believe that you are immune to these postpartum mind games, think again. Just the numbers alone should be enough to change your mind. Three million new moms get the baby blues and more than 500,000 (perhaps closer to one million) come down with full-blown postpartum depression each year! How many millions of you will have the baby blahs?

It is important for you to face these issues squarely, and not play Russian roulette with your emotions and body chemistry. You see, there is only one person who can take control of your mental and physical well-being. It's not a family member, friend, or health professional. It's *you!*

KEEP YOUR MOOD UP AND YOUR DRESS SIZE DOWN

Think of yourself right now. Your spirits may be dampened. You may lack energy and sleep, and this pattern may continue for months because many of your hormones (including serotonin and your sexual hormones) function according to specific day-night cycles that are being interrupted by your lack of sleep. It's time for a quick change.

RESTORE YOURSELF!

In the first few weeks and months following the birth of your child, your body will be restoring itself with the food that you eat. Your pregnancy was a wonderful, enriching experience that gave you a lot. It also took away a lot, and your body after delivery is not the same as it was before conception. Did you ever wonder how your baby developed its skeleton? Simple. It leached the calcium from *your* bones and *your* diet. Every cell in your baby's body came from either your food or from your body itself, and this pattern continues if you breast-feed.

No wonder you feel so out of kilter. Besides all the hormonal changes that we have been discussing, you are probably depleted of many vital nutrients, vitamins, and minerals. The foods that you eat now will go a long way toward reviving and energizing you. But before you rush to restore yourself by what you eat, be certain of one thing: The real secret to weighing less than before you were pregnant is to reinforce your mind/body connection and kiss the baby blahs good-bye.

This you can do by restoring your normal level of serotonin.

Many women with severe postpartum depression require prescription medications to restore their serotonin levels. There is a class of antidepressants called *selective serotonin reuptake inhibitors* (SSRIs) that do just that. Examples of SSRIs include Prozac, Zoloft, and Paxil. These medications work by altering the metabolism of serotonin in the brain so that the cerebral level of serotonin remains higher than normal. Having higher levels of serotonin, as you have learned, puts you in a better mood, allows you to sleep better, fights fatigue, and allows the natural weight loss process we have been discussing to proceed without a hitch. Certainly, these medications are a godsend for those of you with severe postpartum depression. I can't tell you how many new moms suffering from severe postpartum depression have had their lives changed by taking the proper antidepressant medication. If you or someone you know is suffering with severe postpartum depression, seek professional help as soon as possible.

The vast majority of new moms, however, will experience the less severe form of postpartum depression, the baby blahs, and nature lets you raise your level of serotonin without medication. In fact, nature allows you to eat your way out of the baby blahs, shrinking your mind and body at the same time! Here's how.

SEROTONIN BUILDING: DO IT YOURSELF

Serotonin is a protein and, like all proteins, it is composed of small building blocks called *amino acids*. There are over twenty different amino acids, but the one that your brain needs to make serotonin is called *tryptophan*. Tryptophan is the rarest of all the amino acids, and since your body cannot manufacture it, all of your tryptophan comes from the protein in foods that you eat, such as eggs, meat, fish, and soy. Protein begets protein.

When your brain has more tryptophan at its disposal, it makes more serotonin. The problem is that traffic into the brain can get congested because other amino acids are trying to get in at the same time, and tryptophan, as the rarest of all the amino acids, is at the back of the line. A few years ago, Drs. Judith and Richard Wurtman discovered that there is one food that can actually push tryptophan to the front of the line, and one hormone that can then squeeze tryptophan into your brain to create more serotonin. This in turn elevates your mood, helps you sleep, and of course helps you lose weight. This mind-altering food is the underappreciated and often-maligned *carbohydrate*, and the serotonin-boosting hormone is *insulin*.

FOOD FOR THOUGHT

Carbohydrates, or "carbs," are the starches and sugars in bread, pasta, rice, corn, potatoes, grains, honey, lactose (milk sugar), fruits, and table sugar.

After you eat a carbohydrate-containing meal, the level of your blood sugar goes up. This causes your pancreas to secrete the hormone insulin, which is involved in all phases of carbohydrate metabolism. Insulin, it was discovered, also pushes tryptophan from your blood into your brain, where it is used to make serotonin. Since protein and fat do not cause insulin to be secreted by the pancreas, they do not cause tryptophan to enter the brain; only carbohydrates do! But all carbohydrates are not equal serotonin builders.

There are two types of carbohydrates: simple and complex. Simple carbohydrates are sugars such as glucose and fructose. Combinations of simple carbohydrates make up everything from table sugar to pancake syrup, corn syrup, and honey. These sugars put the "sweet" in our sweets. From sodas, cakes, and candy to ice cream and sports drinks, they all taste so good and so sweet because of their simple sugar content, usually dominated by fructose, one of the sweetest sugars.

Complex carbohydrates, on the other hand, are starches that are so named because they have more complex molecular structures than simple sugars. Complex carbohydrates are superior to simple sugars at building serotonin. Fructose, for example, does *nothing* to help synthesize serotonin. Complex carbohydrates found in starches like pasta, whole wheat bread, grains, rice, potatoes, beans, peas, oatmeal, barley, and corn are the serotonin builders that your brain needs.

Just about everyone loves complex carbohydrates. Food surveys conducted nationwide consistently show that the number one food type that women crave is carbohydrates in the guise of bread, rolls, bagels, and crackers. Who doesn't like pasta? Or rice? What about mashed potatoes or corn on the cob? Who can resist a bowl or two of a favorite breakfast cereal? Complex carbohydrates are mouthwateringly delicious in their own right. However, don't lose sight of what they will do for you now: keep your postpartum body on its predestined natural weight loss course.

Complex carbohydrates need only a few hours to raise your serotonin level. By including complex carbohydrates in each meal, you can keep your serotonin level up the whole day. Higher levels of serotonin mean that you are going to be in an upbeat mood, sleep better, have more energy, and of course, lose weight! Now, for your ace in the hole: You don't have to drown in complex carbohydrates to be successful. Emphasizing complex carbohydrates after delivery does not mean that you have to stuff yourself with pasta, bread, or rolls. Far from it! An amazing thing about the postpartum is that, unlike at any other time, your serotonin levels are extremely sensitive to even slight changes in your complex carbohydrate intake. Small changes go a long way now. For instance, having a whole-grain English muffin instead of one made with processed flour, or having some pasta with your steak, can make a huge difference in both your mood and your weight loss!

By the way, it was recently discovered that severe dieting lowers the concentration of tryptophan, which causes a decrease in the level of serotonin. This may explain why women who are on a strict diet seem so unhappy!

Can it really be this simple? Can eating foods containing complex carbohydrates really make such a big difference? Of course it can, but only because after you have given birth, your body's biochemistry has changed so much. Your delivery, in fact, has created a temporary hormonal imbalance that includes a decline in your serotonin levels. This can be countered by doing something as simple as eating pasta, cereal, rice, and potato dishes. Eating complex carbohydrates at any other time except the postpartum will neither raise your mood nor help your weight loss, because your level of serotonin would then be at its normal, higher levels. An exception would be during episodes of premenstrual syndrome. Research has shown that women who suffer from premenstrual syndrome experience fewer symptoms if they eat high complex carbohydrates before their periods.

The postpartum is the perfect time for the perfect food, complex carbohydrates! Keep in mind that lowered levels of serotonin can sometimes make your body crave carbohydrates over other types of food, and we want your body to be happy by giving it what it needs!

THE PERFECT POSTPARTUM FOOD

Beyond their serotonin-raising ability, complex carbohydrates are the perfect postpartum food for other reasons. Besides helping with weight loss and putting you in the proper postpartum mind-set, complex carbohydrates can also help you navigate some of the land mines of the first trimester of weight loss. That's why I call complex carbohydrates the "perfect postpartum food." I believe that there are five criteria for the perfect postpartum food, and complex carbohydrates fulfill them all:

1. **The Perfect Food Must Be Easy to Prepare:** This is hardly the time for gourmet cooking. You are tired and stressed, and spending a lot of time in the kitchen is not for you. Pouring a bowl of breakfast cereal or having some peanut butter and jelly on whole wheat bread doesn't seem too taxing! If you have to prepare meals for your family, then pasta and rice dishes, for example, are among the easiest things to make. Husbands, boyfriends, and other family members can easily help, even if it's only to boil the water!

2. **The Perfect Food Should Provide Necessary Nutrition:** Complex carbohydrates provide your body with ample energy calories that you can use right now. Many complex carbohydrates are excellent sources of protein and in fact are often the main source for vegetarians and vegans. In addition, they can be a good source of vitamins, which your postpartum body needs for restoration.

3. **The Perfect Food Provides Energy for Your Muscles:** Even carrying an 8-pound baby makes your muscles work! What food do marathon runners load up on before a competition to make their muscles perform optimally? Complex carbohydrates! Unlike fat or protein, only they can power muscles with instant energy, the same kind of energy that you need right now.

4. **The Perfect Food Fights Constipation:** Constipation can be a big nuisance after delivery. Many complex carbohydrates are high in fiber, and fiber promotes normal bowel movements.

5. **The Perfect Food Must Taste Good:** Pasta, rice, bread, or rolls, anyone?

DON'T BE A FATHEAD

Before we go any further, let's lay to rest the eternal diet debate: Which diet is best for weight loss? High fat? High protein? Low carbohydrate? It seems that we all have our own views and champion our own diet guru. It's time to come together and use common sense and a scale once more.

The postpartum period is unique. Your new understanding of the hormonal changes that your body has undergone should alter the way you approach your food intake. Even though some of you may have lost weight temporarily in the past by following a high-fat or high-protein diet, trying one of these fad diets in the postpartum can be disastrous. You will totally negate what your body and you are trying to work on together: fostering your mind/body connection and losing weight. A high-protein or high-fat diet will sabotage the extraordinary weight loss conditions that your body has established for you.

SAY NO TO HIGH PROTEIN, FOUR TIMES

Eating a high-protein diet after delivery will block your weight loss efforts, especially if you are overweight. There are four reasons why high-protein diets are wrong for you in the postpartum:

1. **Protein Closes the Brain to Serotonin:** Having too much protein in your system interferes with your ability to make serotonin, because it blocks the transport of tryptophan into your brain. Unlike carbohydrates, protein does not cause insulin to be secreted by the pancreas. Without insulin, tryptophan is stranded in the bloodstream and never gets the chance to enter your brain. Also, protein is made up of other amino acids, which tend to compete with tryptophan. The more excess protein you eat, the more competing amino acids in your blood block tryptophan from entering the brain.

2. **High Protein—Are You Kidneying Me?** Protein from your food that is not utilized by your body is processed by your kidneys. The kidneys can handle a finite amount of protein. Exceeding this level just makes your kidneys work overtime. During pregnancy, your kidneys had to work harder than usual to help filter all the extra waste products, including those from protein that would otherwise accumulate harmfully in both you and your baby. After delivery, your kidneys are tired but still have to work hard, like the other parts of your body, in order to restore themselves. Too much protein now taxes your kidneys. Don't your kidneys deserve a break? Let them rest!

3. **High Protein, High Fat:** A high-protein diet is really a high-fat diet. With the exception of soy, some fish, and skim milk products, almost all protein sources—such as meat, cheese, and peanuts—are fat-laden as well. Even a skinless fillet of chicken breast is 20 percent fat! No matter how hard you try, you will automatically eat more fat when you try a high-protein diet, unless you are a strict vegetarian.

4. **High Protein, Low Calcium:** There is scientific evidence that high protein intake interferes with the way that calcium is metabolized in the body, making calcium levels in the blood fall. Since calcium is one of the nutrients that new moms are most deficient in, now is not the time to upset the calcium balance in your body. It may lead to thinning of your bones, or *osteoporosis*, which can cause bone fractures later in life.

SAY NO TO HIGH FAT, SEVEN TIMES

If you think that eating a high-protein diet in the postpartum will give you problems, just look at what a high-fat diet will do for you now: nothing but clog your system and sabotage the works. Not just one way, but seven ways! Count them, seven!

1. **Fat Can Be a Big Diet Downer:** There is a chemical in your brain called *galanin*. High-fat meals turn galanin "on" like a light switch. When galanin is activated, it competes with and overruns serotonin. You then feel tired, depressed, and hungry. This is not what you want or what you need. You end up fighting your body, and you already know who is going to win that battle!

2. **Fat Fights Fat Loss, Part I:** As we mentioned on page 30, leptin is your very own fat-melting hormone. You will become very familiar

with it in the next weight loss trimester because it is the key hormone for success for all overweight new moms (Type B's). Eating too much fat now can overwhelm your own fat-melting hormone, literally smothering your ability to burn fat.

3. **Fat Fights Fat Loss, Part II:** Fat enzymes are your body's laborers, pushing fat into fat cells. During pregnancy, your fat enzymes became superactive, working overtime to help you put on fat. In the first trimester of weight loss, levels of these enzymes fall, and they "sleep" for a few weeks. Eating high-fat foods wakes them up. Do you really want to do that?

4. **Fat, the Thyroid Slayer:** Research suggests that high fat consumption can depress the proper functioning of your thyroid gland, the gland at the base of your neck which controls your metabolism. After delivery, some women experience a sluggish thyroid that can actually cause a syndrome that mimics postpartum depression and causes weight gain. As you can see, the thyroid gland has enough of its own problems after delivery without having to worry about being flooded with fatty foods. Don't mess with your thyroid!

5. **Fat Begets Fat:** While you were pregnant, the levels of fats in your blood such as cholesterol and triglycerides rose dramatically. This is considered a natural development of pregnancy, and the levels return to normal by themselves after delivery if left unmolested. Of course, if you are a woman with the genetic predisposition to developing what is popularly known as hardening of the arteries (*atherosclerosis*), then the last thing you would want to do is eat high-fat foods now, keeping your blood levels of cholesterol and triglyceride at their pregnancy levels. By doing this you are theoretically activating the atherosclerotic process that would put you at lifelong risk of developing heart disease.

6. **Fat Begets Fatigue:** One of the most common complaints that women have in the weeks and sometimes months after delivery is a diminished energy level. High-fat meals do not help. Studies show that high-fat meals cause drowsiness, explaining your desire to sleep after a high-fat dinner, for instance. In addition, your body needs energy right now, on a day-to-day basis. Fat, as a stored form of energy, does not supply the immediate energy that your muscles need.

7. **Fat Makes No Sense:** This is my personal favorite reason for not eating a diet high in fat. Eating fat defies common sense, and it will defy your scale! Common sense leads us to ask: If you are trying to get rid of fat from your body, why take more aboard at this crucial time? More fat

in means less fat out! Female bodybuilders who know and understand their bodies "to the max" always limit their fat intake before a contest to "cut up" or lose the fat over their muscles. Aren't you in the bodybuilding business yourself, now, as you try to shed fat and sculpt yourself?

We recommend no high-protein, no high-fat, no "high-" anything except for the way you feel about yourself. Your body is searching for balance, and so should you. Moderation rules. The right postpartum combination of complex carbohydrates, proteins, and fats will keep your mind/body connection strong and healthy, and promote your body's natural postpartum ability to shed fat.

EATING FOR POSTPARTUM WEIGHT LOSS SUCCESS

Choices, choices, choices. You had to make many important decisions over the past few months and will continue to do so. From deciding where to deliver, which doctor to use, and whether or not to breast-feed, and on to the name you picked for your new baby, you hope you made all the right choices with as little left to chance as possible. You want to lose as much weight as you can now, so you already have made a very smart decision: not to leave your post-pregnancy weight loss to chance either. You already know that complex carbohydrates, protein, and fat are the crux of a balanced eating plan during the first weight loss trimester. Once again you need choices: smart, healthy, quality food choices, like the ones in the *Hello, Baby! Good-bye, Baby Fat!* eating and lifestyle plan.

These days, it seems like everyone wants to understand their food intake in terms of percentages of protein, fat, and carbohydrates. The first question people ask about new diets is how much fat, protein, and carbohydrates diets allow. Some low-fat diets, for example, limit daily fat calorie intake to 10 percent, while high-fat diets allow more than 50 percent fat calories per day! Some high-protein diets consist of almost 60 percent protein! During the first trimester of weight loss, you should be eating between 50 to 60 percent complex carbohydrates, 25 to 30 percent fat, and 20 percent protein. Consider this your secret *serotonin-building formula*. Here's why.

Eating a diet containing 50 percent or more complex carbohydrates makes your insulin work more efficiently, which speeds up your weight loss. That's because insulin, as we outlined on page 69, is a serotonin builder. No one knows why you need to keep your complex carbohydrate intake at this high level to make insulin work best, but consider this: Adult-onset diabetics who have trouble with insulin and carbohydrate metabolism are advised to eat a diet consisting of between 50 and 60 percent complex carbohydrates to help their blood sugar problems! Conversely, diets high in fat and lower in carbohydrates have an adverse effect on insulin and can promote weight gain. Pregnant women, especially overweight pregnant women, have lots of insulin floating around in their blood. As you recall, excess insulin favors weight gain by increasing appetite and fat deposits. You have come way too far for that!

Why keep your daily intake of fat between 25 and 30 percent? This range of fat intake appears to be low enough not to gum up serotonin's activity in your brain, as we said before, and high enough to provide your food with good taste. There is no denying that fat tastes good, and we want you to enjoy your food. There is another postpartum reason not to limit your fat too much now: You need dietary fat to help your body restore itself, because fat is an important component of the outer coating of your cells, known as *cell membranes*. A proper fat intake is vital for a nursing mom, because a newborn needs fat for the proper development of his or her nervous system.

Finally, the guideline for consuming 20 percent protein is based on a simple physiological fact: Your body composition is 20 percent protein! No matter how much protein you ingest, you never exceed that 20 percent. The *Hello, Baby! Good-bye, Baby Fat!* eating and lifestyle plan provides plenty of protein for nursing and non-nursing new moms.

YOU, THE VIRTUAL DIETICIAN

Your postpartum body requires balance. Beginning on page 188 you will find two weeks' worth of menu suggestions for the first trimester of weight loss and beyond. These core menus are based on the principles of postpartum nutritional balance outlined above, and they amplify your postpartum body's ability to lose weight. The food plan provides the right amount of complex carbohydrates to allow you to raise your serotonin levels, and enough fat and protein to ensure a smooth and healthy postpartum weight loss experience. Since you are essentially rebuilding your body, and since protein is your body's building block, we take no chances with protein allowances. Breast-feeding women secrete between 5 and 10 grams of protein a day in their milk, so they need to ingest an extra 12 grams of protein every day. I also believe that non-breast-feeding women have an increased need for protein to rebuild their body, and the usual recommendation that they ingest 65 grams of protein per day is too low. Therefore, the protein content of the core menu averages about 75 grams a day, which is ideal for all new moms, nursing or not. Recommended sources of protein include low-fat dairy products, fish, egg whites, chicken, turkey, and lean-cut beef. Avoid luncheon meats and cold cuts: They contain too much fat and preservatives!

With the core menus you get to eat "real food" like pasta, cereal, rice, and potatoes along with fish, meat, and chicken. In fact, many of the food suggestions are listed by brand name to show that you have easy access to this type of eating. There are no celery sticks or rice cakes on this plan! (Those of you who are vegetarians or vegans can of course eat lots of complex carbohydrates, eschew the animal protein choices, and substitute soy and tofu instead.) The way of eating outlined in these core menus is healthy for other family members as well.

Each day's breakfast, lunch, and dinner all appear on one page for convenience's sake. The total calorie count and percentages of carbo-hydrates, fat, and protein appear on the bottom of each page, making it easy for you to see what kind of nutrition you will need, both quali-tatively and quantitatively, to become the next postpartum weight loss success story. On the page facing each menu, you will find a weight loss companion page filled with fun facts and inspirational quotations about food and life. I hope they enrich your weight loss experience!

The core menus contain between 1500 and 1700 calories for non-nursing moms (and between 1800 and 2100 calories for breast-feeding moms). The reason for this variation is simple. You are not a robot, and in real life you tend not to eat the same amount of food each day. Notice that nursing moms really don't need much more food than non-nursing moms; they require only about 250 to 350 extra calories per day.

Although the idea behind these core menus is for you not to have to count every calorie, staying within these calorie ranges is important. Unlike at any other time in your life, you are trying to accomplish three things with your food intake now. First, you need to take in enough calories to help your body to repair itself while also allowing for weight loss. Second, if you are nursing, you need extra nutrition to support your baby's development. Third, you need to ingest the proper amount of complex carbohydrates to keep your serotonin level up. The core menus were designed with these three guidelines in mind.

I've told you that I don't believe in diets. The core menus have only two weeks' worth of suggestions, so you will be on your own the rest of the time. That's the way that it should be! Try following the core menus for the first two weeks, and see how easy it is! The core menus should be used as templates from which you can form the new eating habits that will ensure your success. Reviewing tomorrow's food intake the night before is one way to help reinforce your sense of control. You become your own best dietician! The easiest way to begin your new career is by purchasing one of the many nutrition counters that list foods by their brand names. It becomes easy to make the right choices once you know the carbohydrate, fat, and protein content of everything you eat.

The core menus are trying to teach you something else besides balanced postpartum nutrition. They're inculcating a sense of portion size. A Type A (desirable-weight) new mom may look at these menus and think that they provide too much food. A Type B (overweight) or Type C (obese) new mom may think there is not enough food. It has been demonstrated that overweight women tend to *underestimate* their portion sizes and total calorie intake by 50 percent! Portion control can be learned only with practice, and portion control is the key to long-term weight loss. What better time to start than now, when your appetite is naturally decreased? No matter what you weigh, you will have to discover what portion size works best for you, using common sense and a scale. If weight loss is proceeding too slowly, cut back on your portion sizes or cut back on the three daily built-in snacks. If you are losing weight but are still hungry, increase the portion sizes.

When you begin to make your own food choices, be sure to plug them into the postpartum serotonin-building formula contained in the core menus. If you do this and pay attention to the portion sizes, you can't go wrong. Here is a list of the serotonin-raising complex carbohydrates that you can use in planning your future meals. Make certain that the portion sizes of these foods are consistent with those of the core menus.

COMPLEX CARBOHYDRATES THAT RAISE SEROTONIN

1. **Cereals,** cooked: wheat, rice, oatmeal. Ready-to-eat: shredded wheat, bran or corn flakes, puffed rice, whole-grain. Avoid sugar-filled children's breakfast cereals at all costs.

2. **Pasta:** Any pasta is suitable; just keep your sauces to the basic tomato sauce or a pat of margarine. Avoid grated cheeses.

3. **Breads:** Whole wheat and whole grain are best. Avoid all refined-flour white breads, rolls, and bagels. Crackers are OK.

4. **Rice:** white or brown

5. **Wheat germ**

6. **Legumes:** beans, peas, lentils, peanuts

7. **Starchy vegetables:** corn, potatoes

There are certain complex carbohydrates to avoid because they contain too many simple sugars and fat to be of any use to you now. These include: cornbread and any fried carbohydrate, like french fries or fried rice.

Many complex carbohydrates are excellent sources of protein. These include grains (pasta, cereals, and whole wheat bread), legumes (soybeans, tofu, kidney beans, peanuts, lentils), and nuts. Keep in mind that complex carbohydrates do not supply the body with complete proteins. If you are a vegetarian or vegan, be sure you know the amino acid breakdown of the foods that you eat so you can consume foods that help your body synthesize protein.

A HANDS-DOWN FAVORITE

As a new mother, you won't have time to measure each portion of every food you eat. You don't have to! Do what the pros do: Learn to eyeball your food portions by visualizing suitable portions as everyday objects with which you are familiar. For instance, a serving of any solid main dish should be the size of two tennis balls. A side dish serving should be roughly the size of one tennis ball. A deck of cards is the same size as three ounces of fish or meat. A tablespoon of peanut butter or jelly is the size of a walnut. An ounce of cheese is the size of a large marble.

Another technique is the so-called "hand rule." Look at your hand. Your palm is the size of a three-ounce portion of meat. A portion of complex carbohydrates such as pasta should fit, even if piled, into your palm. Make a fist. That's the size of one cup of anything! One ounce of anything is about the size of your thumb!

Still another way to learn portion control, and probably the easiest way, is called the "fill-your-plate" rule. Since each meal that you eat should contain at least 50 percent complex carbohydrates, fill up half your plate with rice, pasta, mashed potatoes, or corn, for instance. The rest of your plate should be filled with protein, vegetables, and fruit. By the way, you can have as many vegetables as you want, but fruit should be limited to two pieces per day because fruits contain simple sugars that provide extra calories without raising your serotonin level.

THE SNACK CLAUSE

The core menus contain three snacks per day! After all, everyone loves to snack. For those of you who must have your chocolate bars, cake and ice cream, listen to this: It's OK to exchange 300 calories of your favorite snack for three of the recommended snacks on the menus. But please snack with these three points in mind:

• Be sure to substitute, and not add, your snack calories for the snacks in the menus.
• Do not exceed 300 total calories from your snacks per day.
• Be certain to finish your snack before 8:00 P.M. This is extremely important, as you will learn shortly.

If you still need more to satisfy your snacking urges, here is a short list of quickie snacks, all of which contain *less* than 50 calories!

UNDER-50-CALORIE "QUICKIE SNACKS"

• 1 ounce raisins—48 calories!
• 1 cup of air-popped popcorn—30 calories!
• 11 jelly beans—44 calories!
• 1 small nonfat cappuccino—45 calories!
• 1 cup of strawberries—45 calories!

And here is a short list of snacks containing less than 100 calories:

UNDER-100-CALORIE "QUICKIE SNACKS"

- 1 low-fat Granola bar (Kellogg's)—80 calories!
- 2 slices of fresh pineapple—90 calories!
- 8 saltines (Premium)—96 calories!
- 10 baked potato chips (Lay's)—100 calories!
- 50 mini-pretzels (Keebler)—65 calories!

SUCCESS AT LAST!

The first question everyone asks is, "How much weight will I lose?" Following the eating format of the core menus should enable any non-nursing Type A (desirable-weight) new mom to lose at least one to two pounds a week or more. This means that the average Type A new mom should be able to lose all her weight by the end of this trimester with little difficulty. If you are a Type B (overweight) or Type C (obese) new mom, your weight loss will get off to a good start and you will lose even more weight per week than Type A moms! However, since you probably won't be able to lose all your weight during the first trimester of weight loss, your efforts need to be continued into the next weight loss trimester. Again, let me emphasize that nursing moms have a different pattern of weight loss. Turn to Chapter Eight for more information.

DETAILS COUNT!

The best thing about this meal plan is that it's short! The first trimester of weight loss lasts just ninety days. That is not even enough time to get bored with the selections, unless you find weight loss itself boring! After the first two weeks, you can repeat the menus and start substituting your own foods. Just remember to stay within the 1500 to 1700 calorie range (1800 to 2100, if you nurse) and stick with the postpartum serotonin-building formula of over 50 percent carbohydrates, slightly less than 30 percent fat, and 20 percent protein.

If you feel up to it, you can try some of the delicious recipes provided by Katy Champ, a gourmet and health-conscious cook who has successfully lost all of her pregnancy weight and then some—not once, but twice!

Don't be afraid to try new things. Experiment. Any pasta dish that you make that is not smothered in butter or fat-containing sauces is fine. Ditto for rice or bean dishes. Be liberal with your vegetables and your whole wheat breads, but not with butter or margarine.

How you prepare your food is important, too. A piece of chicken, for example, can be ruined for you if it is fried or cooked in grease. Here is a list of cooking methods that help keep the fat out of your postpartum life.

THE BEST LOW-FAT COOKING METHODS

- Bake
- Roast
- Broil
- Microwave
- Steam
- Grill
- Stir-fry

If your food is not prepared using one of the methods on this list, avoid it!

Finally, a few words about alcohol. Alcohol is a depressant, and as such, it has a negative effect on serotonin. You want to avoid anything that will interfere with restoring your serotonin level and function. Two or three drinks per week are probably the maximum. If you drink more than that, you will sabotage your body's weight loss efforts. Keep in mind that alcohol contains about 7 calories a gram, almost double the amount in regular carbohydrates (4 calories per gram), and right up there with fat at 9 calories per gram. Breast-feeding moms should not drink alcohol, period.

After only a few days of eating according to the menu plans, you will not only find that your dress size is shrinking, but your mood will improve, you will have more energy, and you will enjoy the postpartum period the way that you should.

POSTPARTUM FAST-FOOD DELIGHT

Recognizing that many postpartum women will be visiting fast-food restaurants, we have devoted Chapter Eleven to helping you make the healthiest choices possible. You can eat fast food and still keep the postpartum weight loss cause alive once you learn the calorie counts and fat content of each food choice. We have broken down the menus of the top national fast-food chains to enable you to do just that. I hope that you also enjoy two fun lists that we have compiled for you: *The Best of Fast Food* and *The Worst of Fast Food*.

Now it's time to fine-tune your first trimester of weight loss eating habits and increase your chances to weigh less than before pregnancy.

FOUR WAYS TO FINE-TUNE YOUR EATING

1. **Timing Is Everything, Mom:** To be in complete sync with your body during the first trimester, you should avoid eating past 7:30 or 8:00 P.M. Nothing. Not an apple, a cracker, a cookie, a vegetable, or that bowl of popcorn. Nothing. The reason? It's all about metabolism. Your metabolism undergoes changes over a 24-hour period. In fact, it has its own sleep-wake cycle. During the day your metabolism rises. It then begins to fall at about 7:30 to 8:00 P.M. This makes perfect sense because during the day, when you are active, you need a more rapid metabolism to provide you with energy. At night while you sleep, you don't. It seems that whenever your metabolism slows, enzymes that deposit fat become more active. Remember that we said that the chief enzyme for depositing fat, fat lipase, is far less active in the immediate postpartum period? Let's keep it that way! Eating at night when your metabolism has slowed will wake up this enzyme and make it easy for any excess food that you eat to stick to your thighs and hips in the form of stored fat. Now, suppose you go out to dinner. Go earlier, and go complex carbohydrate! For you overweight new moms there is an even more important reason to observe this 8:00 P.M. food curfew. In Chapter Seven you will discover how going to sleep on an empty stomach will help you help leptin, your own fat-melting hormone, keep your weight off forever!

2. **Take Your Vitamins, Mom:** There is one surefire way to gain weight, and that is to try to get all the necessary vitamins you need from your food alone. Of course you want to replace any vitamins and minerals that you are missing from their most natural source, your food. However, there is one huge problem that your doctor or nutritionist may not have told you about. There is *no* way you can fulfill the Recommended Dietary Allowance (RDA) for each nutrient through your food intake alone, and still lose weight. In fact, if you follow the current guidelines,

you will gain weight! That's because the food needed to get all of your required nutrients adds up to over 2700 calories a day! Keep in mind that these RDAs represent the minimum amounts of nutrients that you need, *not* the optimum amounts for health. Let's look at calcium, for example. During pregnancy, you lost calcium. Breast-feeding women lose even more. The RDA for calcium for a breast-feeding woman is 1200 milligrams per day. It is estimated that the average woman consumes 500 milligrams from her diet. Where is the rest supposed to come from? Milk is the best food source for calcium, but how much milk can an adult woman drink each day? What about getting it from another dairy product, such as cottage cheese? It turns out that cottage cheese is a poor source of calcium: You would have to eat four pounds of cottage cheese per day to fulfill your daily calcium requirement!

What about magnesium? The recommended daily dose is 320 milligrams, but the average diet contains about 200 milligrams. Where do you get the other 120 milligrams per day? One of the best food sources for magnesium is wheat germ. You need about three-quarters of a cup of wheat germ each day to get the proper amount. When is the last time you had almost a cup of wheat germ? Could *you* do it every day?

Did you know that zinc is an important mineral for pregnant and breast-feeding women? You need about 15 milligrams per day. The best food source for zinc is oysters. *Oysters?* Next comes amaranth, a grain. You have to eat almost three cups to get your daily recommended amount. Three cups? I don't even know what amaranth is! Low-fat yogurt also contains zinc, but you would need seven yogurts a day to get your daily fix of zinc. We could go on and on, especially when you consider that each day a new mom, nursing or not, has to ingest sixty different nutrients from her food to maintain her health and that of her baby!

There are two obvious points here. First, if you want to fulfill the RDA for all your nutrients and still lose weight, you need to take vitamin and mineral supplements. You took them before you were pregnant and during your pregnancy, and taking them a few more months is no big hassle. Second, you are using these vitamin and mineral supplements to complement, not replace, your food intake, and that's the healthy way to get *all* the minerals and vitamins you need without sacrificing your health or your ability to lose weight. Supplements, of course, contain no calories. Enjoy your food, and remember that eating is supposed to be a pleasurable experience. Don't analyze every aspect of your food to see what its mineral or vitamin content is; that's overkill!

Here is a list of the RDAs for the vitamins and minerals that post-partum women need. Notice that the requirements for nursing women are quite different from those for non-nursing moms.

Essential Postpartum Vitamins and Minerals

NUTRIENT	RDA FOR NON-BREAST-FEEDING MOM	RDA FOR BREAST-FEEDING MOM
Vitamin A	800 mcg RE (retinol equivalents)	1,300 mcg RE (retinol equivalents)
Vitamin D	5 mcg	10 mcg
Vitamin E	8 mg	12 mg
Vitamin K	65 mcg	65 mcg
Vitamin C	60 mg	95 mg
Thiamine	1.1 mg	1.6 mg
Riboflavin	1.3 mg	1.8 mg
Niacin	15 mg	20 mg
Vitamin B_6	1.6 mg	2.1 mg
Folic acid	180 mcg*	280 mcg*
Vitamin B_{12}	2 mcg	2.6 mcg
Calcium	1000 mg	1200 mg
Phosphorous	800 mg	1200 mg
Magnesium	280 mg	355 mg
Iron	15 mg	15 mg
Zinc	12 mg	19 mg
Iodine	150 mcg	200 mcg
Selenium	55 mcg	75 mcg

*As of 1997, it is recommended that women of childbearing age consume 400 mcg of folic acid.

These RDAs are, in my opinion, too low, especially for women who are breast-feeding. Prescription prenatal vitamins and many over-the-counter high-potency vitamin formulas contain more of the nutrients that you need. Many new moms—especially if they are nursing—are advised to continue taking their prenatal vitamins in the postpartum, and I agree with this practice.

Make certain to check with your health professional before you take any vitamin or mineral supplement.

Now here's a quick two-minute vitamin course that will help you lose weight, increase your mood and energy, and sleep better.

There are two B complex vitamins that help serotonin do its job, pantothenic acid and inositol. Pantothenic acid is found in meat, chicken, sunflower seeds, and legumes. Inositol is found in citrus fruits and complex carbohydrates. They both help your brain's neurotransmitters (such as serotonin) function properly. By adding a vitamin B complex supplement (that is water-soluble), you can safely increase your pantothenic acid quota to 25 milligrams from the 5 milligrams that are usually found in multivitamin supplements. Inositol is found in lecithin capsules, which are available in any health store. Take one per day, preferably before sleep.

Folic acid also helps combat depression and can increase energy. You may take a folic acid supplement or it may included in your B vitamin complex supplement. Doses up to 400 micrograms, which is the new recommended dose, are known to be safe. You should know that as of January 1998, all enriched grain cereals sold in the United States contain an extra 140 micrograms of folic acid per 100 grams of cereal.

Finally, zinc is a mineral that theoretically helps serotonin function better. Zinc is known to be present in high concentrations in the brain. A zinc supplement that doubles your recommended daily allowance from 12 to 25 milligrams is suggested.

3. **Caffeine-Free, Mommy.** Limit your caffeine intake during the first weight loss trimester. It would be great if you could avoid all caffeine-containing drinks, but I am a realist. The average American woman drinks about 30 gallons of caffeinated drinks per year! Caffeine poses obvious problems for breast-feeding moms who don't want to pass this stimulant to the baby via their milk, but we have other concerns, too. Caffeine has been shown to cause mood swings in postpartum women by upsetting the delicate balance between estrogen, progesterone, and serotonin. You certainly don't want to do that! Caffeine can also compromise your already-altered sleep patterns. Any new mom welcomes sleep, and caffeine can decrease not only the amount but the quality of the sleep you get. Establishing regular sleep patterns is important in keeping your mood up, so

limit your caffeine intake. A high caffeine intake also can cause your body to lose potassium, and you don't need that because potassium is important in the body's postpartum self-restoration project.

Everyone knows that coffee, certain teas, and soft drinks contain caffeine, but you may be surprised to find how many other things that we put in our mouths have caffeine in them too. For instance, certain over-the-counter and prescription medications contain caffeine, especially migraine headache and muscle-relaxant medications.

Having the equivalent of two cups of coffee (or about 300 milligrams of caffeine) should probably be your daily limit. Anything more may pose a hazard to your mental health and your weight loss.

Keep in mind that many new moms experience increased thirst for the first few weeks after delivery. This is due to hormonal changes both in the brain and in the glands above the kidneys, called the adrenal glands. Don't fuel your increased thirst with caffeine-containing drinks. Have plenty of cold water, or seltzer, on hand. Avoid drinking club soda, because it contains too much salt.

Here are a few tables to help you determine your caffeine usage.

A New Mom's Caffeine Counter

CAFFEINE CONTENT: BEVERAGES

BEVERAGE (1 CUP)	CAFFEINE (IN MILLIGRAMS)
Coffee, instant	50–150
Coffee, brewed	50–200
Coffee, decaffeinated	1–5
Hot chocolate (cocoa)	2–20
Tea	25–75
Soft drinks (12 ounces):	
Coca-Cola/Diet Coke	46
Diet Pepsi	36
Pepsi One	55
Dr. Pepper/Diet Dr. Pepper	55
Mountain Dew	54

CAFFEINE CONTENT:
NON-PRESCRIPTION DRUGS

NON-PRESCRIPTION DRUG, PER DOSE	CAFFEINE (IN MILLIGRAMS)
Anacin	33
Dexatrim	200!
Excedrin	65
Midol	33
NoDoz	100

Remember that chocolate (especially dark chocolate) and chocolate pudding contain small amounts of caffeine, usually in the range of 5 milligrams per ounce.

4. **Salt of the Earth:** You will also want to watch your salt intake during the first trimester of weight loss. You do not have to severely limit your salt intake; just try not to add lots of table salt to whatever you are eating. Remember that luncheon meats, cold cuts, canned soups, pretzels, pizza, and potato chips are all high in salt. You are watching your salt intake now because excess salt during the first few weeks after delivery can interfere with your mood. Certain parts of your body—including your heart, kidneys, and brain—are very sensitive to the amount of salt you eat Some women are more sensitive to the effects of extra salt than others. While you were pregnant, your body held on to a bit more salt than usual, and this salt retention can persist for a few weeks after delivery. Your body has a built-in mechanism to rid itself of this excess salt. When your salt intake is high, it can depress the function of certain cells in your brain, causing lethargy and headache. Help your mind and body recuperate by limiting your salt intake to the natural salt content of the healthy foods you eat in this first weight loss trimester.

ALTERNATIVE MEDICINE: THREE FOR THE POSTPARTUM

There are three alternative medicines available at most health food stores that may improve your mood and energy level during the first weight loss trimester, and thus indirectly help your weight loss. One, valerian, helps restore your natural sleep patterns; another, dong quai, can give you more energy. Alternative medicines such as these should never be used by nursing moms, because they are passed to the infant via breast milk and their effects on a newborn are totally unknown at this time.

The three herbs that can make a difference now are:

1. **Valerian:** A naturally occurring herb, valerian promotes the onset of sleep. Unlike many prescription and over-the-counter sleep aids, valerian is non-sedating, and you will not get the usual "morning hang-over" associated with these medications. In addition, valerian is non-addictive. The problem with valerian, like other herbs, is that the extracts are not standardized and so the exact dose necessary for sleep is unknown. Find a reputable herbalist in your community and discuss your dosing options with him or her.

2. **Kava:** Kava is an herb derived from the root of a type of pepper plant that grows in the South Pacific region. Like valerian, it posseses tranquilizing properties and can help with sleep. Data to support the use of kava in reducing anxiety and as a sleep aid were presented at a recent meeting of the American Psychiatric Association. It is nonaddictive and is already being used extensively in Europe. It can be brewed like tea, and commercial preparations are already available in health food stores.

3. **Dong quai:** A traditional Chinese herb, dong quai is associated with increased energy levels. Interestingly, this herb contains high concentrations of phytoestrogens, plant substances that act like natural estrogens. Dong quai, therefore, can not only give you more energy, but it can help restore your period and relieve some of the mood alterations of postpartum depression, because a relative lack of estrogen, as you know, helps to explain many of the symptoms of postpartum depression. Some doctors have even experimented with treating postpartum depression with estrogen patches. Dong quai may be the natural alternative. Again, the exact dose needed to garner dong quai's effects is unknown, so check with an herbalist who has experience with dong quai.

EXERCISE, ANYONE? . . . ANYONE?

You do not have to exercise to lose weight in the postpartum. This statement is based on two facts. First, as we stated on page 18, studies show that exercise has no influence on weight loss after delivery. Second, the majority of women I interviewed who eventually lost the most weight postpartum did *not* exercise. Those of you who like to exercise, and who have obtained permission to continue from your doctors, please do so! Exercise has many other health benefits to offer besides weight loss.

However, what is the one thing that new moms need and can never get enough of? Give up? Why, it's toning, of course!

KEGELS, ANYONE?

To get into super shape quickly after delivery, you don't need a glider, a rider, a strider, or a roller. Even with all of your new weight loss there are still certain areas of your body that require extra attention because of the drastic changes they underwent while you were pregnant. These areas need to be toned! Some of you, for various medical or emotional reasons, may not be able right now to follow the toning program that we have designed for you. That's fine. Give yourself time, and when you feel you are up to it, turn to page 111 for complete details.

However, there is one important, often-neglected area that does need to be toned right now. These are the internal muscles that surround your sexual organs and your bladder. Together they form the muscles of your pelvic floor. If you wait too long they become lax, and later in life these loose muscles may cause urinary tract problems. Your pelvic floor muscles can be easily whipped into shape by doing one simple exercise, called "Kegels."

First, let's see what kind of shape your pelvic floor muscles are in. Try this simple experiment: While you are urinating, you should be able to voluntarily stop your flow of urine by tightening your muscles. If you did stop the flow, congratulations: You just performed a Kegel! If you can't stop the flow of urine, your pelvic floor muscles need a tune-up. To practice Kegels, give yourself a few seconds a day to practice tensing the muscles around your vagina and anus. You can do them anywhere, anytime, including while you are in the bathroom or sitting in a chair watching television, or even during sex! Each time you do it, count to five and relax, and never hold your breath. Do twenty repetitions each day, and you'll get the muscles of your pelvic floor back in tip-top shape. Kegels can be done right after giving birth, but check with your doctor first. Tighten up for life!

BACK FOR THE FUTURE

I was quite surprised to learn how many new moms suffer back injuries from carrying newborns, who can seem to get heavier almost by the hour. It's hard to enjoy the postpartum and lose weight if you have back pain! Pregnancy changes your center of gravity, especially if you are overweight. Even simple bending and twisting movements have the potential to cause sprains and pains in the first trimester. Since you will be picking up and putting down your newborn an average of one hundred times a day, a short six-point plan developed by Brian Marks, D.C., a chiropractor from North Carolina and an expert in exercise and back problems, can help keep your spine flexible and prevent injuries. The six-point plan should be practiced each time you lift your baby and will soon become second nature to you.

THE SIX-POINT BACK-SAVER PLAN

Each time you pick up your baby:

1. Stand firm in a balanced position, before you lift. Never lift "on the fly" or while pivoting.
2. Bend your knees to begin your lift. Don't bend at the waist; doing so strains the lower back.
3. Let your knees do the lifting. Push off with both feet firmly on the ground.
4. Keep your back straight and balanced as you come up. Try not to arch your back!
5. Always hold the baby as close to you as possible. This lessens low back strain.
6. Always lift twice: Once in your head (think about what you are doing before you do it), and then with your body.

ONE FINAL THOUGHT

The first weight loss trimester is characterized by profound changes in your body chemistry that allow you to lose the most weight of all three weight loss trimesters. If the statistics are right, by the end of the first weight loss trimester, two million new moms will be within 5 pounds of their pre-pregnancy weight. This number represents mostly Type A (desirable-weight) and some Type B (overweight) new moms. If you are part of this group, that means that you only have to lose, on average, another 6 pounds and you will have achieved your goal: You will weigh less than before you were pregnant. If you have more weight to lose, what are you waiting for? Let's move on to the second weight loss trimester!

Chapter Seven

Three to Six Months Postpartum: The Second Trimester of Weight Loss

You made it through the first three months! With each passing day, you are getting thinner and your baby is getting bigger. That's the way it should be. With the baby blues long gone, your strength and stamina are returning. At about three months after delivery many women claim that they are nearly "back to themselves."

The second weight loss trimester begins three months after delivery and is the crucial weight loss trimester for Type B, or overweight, new moms. Even though your weight loss began after delivery, most of the extra fat that you have accumulated during pregnancy will be coming off now. Waiting ahead is the commanding six-month weight loss wall, and you want to lose as much as possible *now* before you come up against it. You have ninety days left to get your weight loss act together. Don't worry—you can achieve your goals! Obese new moms (Type C), especially those who breast-feed, will also lose a great deal of body fat during this three-month period, but their weight loss efforts will likely continue through the next weight loss trimester as well.

A return to work is imminent for many working women during this trimester, and we will have a lot to say about the relationship between working outside the home and weight loss. It's a fascinating subject that affects all women, no matter what they weigh.

Take a look at yourself. There have been some big changes since delivery. Your belly is flatter; your hips and waist are narrower. Your thighs have been deflating, and your facial bones should be emerging from beneath their cover of fat. Other physical milestones have altered your appearance, and they all point to the incredibly elastic body that you have. In the meantime your hormones are rolling up their sleeves and making changes of their own, changes that will once again cause weight loss.

If you had acne during your pregnancy or after delivery, it should be clearing now, thanks to a rise in estrogen and progesterone. Your facial skin and your hair may have gotten darker during pregnancy. This was due to higher-than-normal levels of a hormone called *melanin*, which is responsible for skin and hair pigmentation. Your own natural color should be returning as melanin levels return to normal. Any hair that grew thicker while pregnant will get thinner, and some women actually lose hair now, albeit temporarily. Any stretch marks on your abdomen, buttocks, and thighs should start turning from red to your natural skin tone, since they are partially caused by changes in blood levels of progesterone. If you had a "C-section," the scar on your abdomen can take up to a year to return to your normal skin hue. However, the defining physical milestone of the second weight loss trimester is the return of your menstrual cycle.

Some of you may already have experienced your first period since conception, but up to 75 percent of new moms will have it during this trimester. Of course, this applies only to non-breast-feeding women. Nursing postpones the return of the period. Some women consider this nursing-induced postponement of menses adequate birth control. My advice: *Don't!* Many a baby has been conceived by a breast-feeding woman, so use some other form of contraception that really works!

Indeed, the return of your period is nature's signal that you will be able to conceive again soon. Your ovaries, which manufacture estrogen and progesterone, have been on vacation during your pregnancy. Now they are up and running, and back to pumping out your usual complement of hormones. Your first period since delivery will be somewhat abnormal, and you may notice that your flow is either scanty or perhaps heavier than what you are used to. This is your body trying to fine-tune itself. It shows that your hormones are still not back to normal levels, but they soon will be. As time passes, and the hormones responsible for your monthly cycles are fortifying themselves, *the door to weight loss appears to be closing.* After all, estrogen will soon be doing what it does best: stimulating your appetite. Progesterone will soon be up to its old trick of making it easier to deposit fat on your body. Remember, it was the low levels of these hormones in the immediate postpartum that allowed you to lose weight in the first place. Now, they are on their way back.

Uh-oh! Are your hormones going to oppose your every weight loss move? Are you once more at the mercy of willpower, self-denial, and finding that perfect fad diet? You know how well those have served you in the past!

Quick, you need some sort of a weight loss edge. To get yours, dial the second weight loss trimester emergency number. The answer comes from deep inside your own fat cells. Something has been helping you lose weight from the moment you gave birth, but you never knew about it until now. It's a marvelous, newly discovered weight loss advantage. To find out all about it, you have to "show me the fat."

SHOW ME THE FAT

Touch a part of you where extra fat has accumulated during your pregnancy, probably your breasts, thighs, hips, buttocks, or abdomen. You won't find much on your back, shoulders, or neck. That's because there is a design behind the way fat is deposited on your body. Your body prefers to add and subtract fat in a certain pattern, with some inherited variations. I call this pattern the *Postpartum Weight Loss Pyramid*, because you lose fat first from the narrowest part of your body—your face—and then your weight loss shifts downward, progressing to the widest areas of your body in an orderly manner. After you lose fat in your face, the extra fat from your breasts is shed, followed by the fat in your abdomen and buttocks. Last, and certainly not least, the fat from your thighs comes off. This is not something you have voluntary control over; it just happens. It doesn't matter if you spend a thousand hours in the gym, or none at all—this sequential top-to-bottom weight loss pattern plays out in its own way.

This chain of weight loss, like your weight gain of pregnancy, has its own logic, which I call "fat logic." Understanding how your own body fat operates is the key to getting rid of it! Let's take a brief trip inside your body, and visit the very place where fat lives: the fat cell.

That fleshy mound that you just touched or pinched is not muscle, nor is it ligaments or bone. It's fat. Greasy, oily, slippery fat. There is

THE POSTPARTUM WEIGHT LOSS PYRAMID

The sequence of shedding fat

HEAD

CHEST

ABDOMINALS

HIPS & BUTTOCKS

THIGHS

Fat comes off your body like a pyramid. You lose weight
from the top of your body first (your face), then downward
to the middle (your abdomen), and finally fat is shed
from your hips, buttocks, and thighs.

nothing else like it in the whole universe. Don't get angry with your
fat. Instead, think of it as your body's long-term reminder to you of all
those huge lunches, dinners, and snacks from the past nine months
and before.

Your fat resides in tiny containers called fat cells that are too small
to be seen by the naked eye. You can't feel a fat cell, either. The mushy
feeling you get when you pinch fat is actually thousands and thousands
of individual fat cells congealed and coalesced together like bunches
of grapes. These mats of fat cells are what get sucked out of the body
during a liposuction procedure.

While you were pregnant and stockpiling fat on your hips, thighs,
and buttocks, your fat cells were like little Pac-Men with mouths open,
always hungry for more. Your fat cells can always accommodate any
extra food that hormones (such as insulin) and enzymes (such as fat
lipase) force into them. You can stuff fat cells with so much fat that
they blow up like balloons. The number of fat cells you have is largely,

but not totally, genetically determined. Type C, or obese, moms are born with more fat cells than thinner moms. Some of you have fat cells that are larger and can hold more fat than others! But fat cells have a lot more going for them than just holding fat—*they're alive!*

Your body's fat cells are not like the inert fat that you cut from your steak. Nor are they like the lardy lump of butter that fills the crevices of your English muffin. Your fat cells are alive, as active and vital as any of your heart, brain, or muscle cells. Fat cells perform vital work for you, and as long as you live, they live too. In fact, when you lose weight your fat cells don't disappear; they merely shrink.

Fat cells store your excess food calories, help shield you against the cold weather, manufacture important molecules, help metabolize hormones such as estrogen, and help your body fight infection. Recently, a stunning scientific discovery uncovered an important weight loss secret contained in your fat cells. This secret will be *your* weight loss edge for the second weight loss trimester, and beyond.

MOM, MEET YOUR NEW FAT-BURNING HORMONE

For decades, overweight people have been claiming that their weight difficulties were caused by glandular problems. Somehow, they said, their glands were making them heavy, a claim that scientists dismissed as nonsense. Thanks to new research, it turns out that the scientists were *wrong* for the right reasons, and overweight people were *right* for the wrong reasons! Scientists had been looking exclusively at malfunctions of the thyroid gland or the pituitary gland as the culprits behind obesity, but the scientists had chosen the wrong glands! The gland that they should have been looking at was the fat cell itself! What the researchers didn't realize is that, amazingly, your fat cells can actually signal your brain to eat more or less. Your own fat cells, then, control your appetite!

A few years ago biologists, armed with new technology, discovered that fat cells are actually glands. Remember, glands make hormones, and the hormone that fat cells make is *leptin*. Leptin and the science behind it may be new to you, but don't worry—they're new to everyone. A few years ago this whole discussion would have been impossible; now you are on the cutting edge of weight loss knowledge. *Leptin* comes from the Greek word for "thin," which gives you an idea of what leptin does for you: *It helps you stay thin*. Leptin is also known as the fat-melting hormone. Although much remains to be learned about leptin, this much is clear: Leptin is a major player in the weight loss game. Here's why. Not only does leptin help burn fat and control your appetite and metabolic rate, it also has a large say in your ability to reproduce. As if all this weren't enough, leptin is the hormone that allows you to reset your set point!

If this hormone can do all that, we need to find a way to make it work for you, and as soon as possible. I have good news for you. You don't have to wait years or spend the millions of dollars that pharmaceutical companies spend on research to find how to use leptin for weight loss. If you recently delivered, leptin can help you right now in the second weight loss trimester.

Let's get back to your fat cells. Each fat cell that you have contains genes. Leptin is made by one of the genes in fat cells, which is called, aptly enough, the obesity (ob) gene. Genes are merely pieces of protein called DNA that contain the genetic code that you received from your parents and pass on to your children. The obesity genes contain the genetic code of your fat, and this is why being overweight runs in families: The genetic code for obesity is transferred from one generation to another. If both you and the father of your child are obese, the chances of your baby's being obese are as high as 70 to 80 percent. If only one of you is obese, there is a 40 percent chance that your baby will be obese. If neither of you is obese, your baby's chances dip to only 10 percent! So leptin plays a role in how much body fat both you and your baby will eventually have. Believe it or not, your baby made leptin when he or she was inside of you. That's because everybody makes leptin. From the thinnest runway model to the heaviest weight lifter, every man, woman, and child manufactures leptin. However, how much leptin is made depends on how much body fat you have. The more fat on your body, the more leptin you make.

Women make more leptin than men and probably utilize leptin differently from men. This leptin gender difference is just the edge you need.

When you were pregnant, you ate more than normal, which filled your fat cells with fat. This excess fat "turns on," or activates, the obesity gene inside the fat cell and directs it to manufacture lots of leptin. Leptin then leaves your fat cells and enters your bloodstream, where it circulates throughout your body. Eventually it travels up to and reaches the appetite control center of your brain. Once there, leptin gives your brain a signal that you should stop eating, because your fat cells have accumulated enough fat. This is how leptin helps your brain control your appetite. At least that's what's supposed to happen. Somehow, however, during pregnancy (especially if you are overweight) the leptin message to stop eating is not interpreted properly by your brain, and more and more leptin is needed to put the brakes on your food intake. This phenomenon is called "leptin resistance": your body makes more and more leptin, yet even this increased amount of leptin doesn't do a good job controlling your appetite. Keep in mind that leptin can not only shut down the appetite, but it can also burn fat and raise even the most sluggish metabolism. Helping leptin do a better job is what the second weight loss trimester is all about.

OF MICE AND WOMEN

Leptin has powerful connections to your reproductive system. Do you remember the pair of "super-fat" mice that were paraded on the evening news a few years ago? Their fifteen minutes of fame made them the second-most-famous mouse couple to date, right behind Mickey and Minnie. Their sudden celebrity status was based on the discovery that these super-fat mice were born without the gene (the ob gene) that makes leptin. Without leptin, these mice were unable to stop eating, and they became grotesquely obese. What a way to become famous!

However, within a few days of receiving injections of leptin, these mice became thin again!

Later, scientists were astounded to find that these leptin-deficient mice were not only obese, they were infertile and had slow metabolisms! Somehow leptin raises metabolism *and* plays a role in a woman's ability to conceive. A few weeks after receiving their leptin injections, the mice were able to conceive, and their metabolism increased! Soon afterward, it was discovered that leptin does exactly the same thing in humans: It controls weight and regulates puberty, fertility, menses, and metabolism. But leptin isn't done yet.

Leptin also monitors how much fat you have on your body, and how much energy you expend, and it tells your brain to eat or not eat accordingly. You need a certain amount of leptin in circulation to keep your appetite in check. But remember this about leptin: LEPTIN IS ONE BIG METABOLIC TATTLETALE. Leptin likes to tell the brain how much food you are eating. Rather than monitor your every culinary move, leptin monitors trends, probably over a few days. If you starve yourself with a three-day miracle diet, for instance, and you lose weight too quickly, your fat cells start to shrink and the amount of leptin that your fat cells make drops. When your brain realizes there is less leptin available, it double-crosses you, not only increasing your appetite but also slowing your metabolism, which causes you to eat more and regain any weight that you lost. These dynamics explain diet failures in a nutshell. You are fighting your body, and you are going to lose every time.

Your level of leptin is closely related to the levels of your sexual hormones, estrogen and progesterone. Through a mechanism that is not fully understood, leptin signals your reproductive organs to make more sexual hormones. As leptin levels rise, so do estrogen and progesterone levels. Conversely, as leptin levels fall, so do estrogen's and progesterone's. This explains why very thin women, like marathon runners and anorectics (people lacking appetite), have difficulties with menstruation and with getting pregnant. These women have very little body fat and, quite often, insufficient levels of leptin to signal the reproductive system that all is well. Without the signal from leptin, you cannot have normal menstrual cycles. Likewise, leptin plays a role in very obese women having difficulties with their menses and in getting pregnant. Having too much body fat alters the way in which the body uses leptin and estrogen. There is a definite optimal body weight range in which leptin operates most effectively, and I believe that this range is related to your set point. Stay with me now; *the weight loss payoff is coming.*

RESETTING YOUR SET POINT

Remember Debbie from Chapter One? She is one of the 400,000 women each year who after delivery weigh less than their pre-pregnancy weight. In order for this to be possible, she, like each of the other women, had to overcome her set point. As you know, the set point is the weight that your body loves to stay at. Maria C., a 35-year-old special education teacher from Westchester County, New York, knows all too well about the set point. The athletic mother of one son, she weighed 135 pounds until two years ago when she went through a bitter divorce. Depressed, within six months her weight mushroomed up to 175 pounds. She wanted her old body back and tried to return to her 135-pound figure, though she admitted to herself that she would "take" 145 pounds. She began a high-protein diet and got down to 158 pounds. Despite having lost 17 pounds, Maria became increasingly dejected. Why was she having so much trouble reaching her ideal weight? Because a few months back, when she weighed 168 pounds, Maria attempted to lose weight by following a near-starvation cabbage soup diet that was popular with some of her on-line friends. Yes, she lost weight, but she could not get beyond 158 pounds. We call this invisible barrier the "set point." Surely you know of someone like Maria, or perhaps this syndrome of stalled weight loss has happened to you. Each of us has his or her own set point.

Although it is not known whether there is a specific location for the set point mechanism, it certainly involves leptin and other hormones, along with obesity genes and the appetite control center of the brain. Think of leptin as the great communicator, sending signals from the genes in your fat cells to your appetite control center. All roads that lead to gaining control over your set point begin with leptin: It was Maria's leptin that sent the sabotaging signal to her brain that 158 pounds should be the limit of her weight loss. Your leptin would usually put the brakes on your weight loss too, but the postpartum makes leptin do some strange things that will help you reset your set point and weigh less than before you were pregnant. If you are ever to break through your set point, I believe that it has to happen now, in the second weight loss trimester.

As we have said, your leptin levels stay elevated in your blood throughout your pregnancy. Precisely at delivery, a remarkable thing happens that will occur only at *this* time in your life: Leptin levels plummet before you lose any fat. Ordinarily, leptin levels decline in your blood only after you lose weight because as you lose weight, your fat cells shrink, become less active, and manufacture less leptin. This postpartum fall in your leptin level is all part of your body's ability to reprogram itself and lower your set point, as you shall see shortly.

Leptin also controls your metabolism. When leptin levels rise, so does your metabolism. When leptin levels fall, your metabolism slows. This combination of a drop in leptin and a slowed metabolism causes an increase in your appetite—a big one! (Remember those leptin-deficient mice that couldn't stop eating?) Needless to say, you then regain any lost weight. But now, in the postpartum, and *only* now, your leptin levels fall before you lose any weight and your metabolism remains elevated. This is an unprecedented biological event, an endowment from nature. Without it, you would be ravenously hungry in the postpartum period and have a slower metabolism, making weight loss impossible. But, now, the opposite has occurred. You are less hungry than usual, and you will stay this way until your leptin can orchestrate your next two or three periods. That's when your leptin, estrogen, and progesterone levels return to full strength and your usual appetite and set point pattern reassert themselves.

This special time period when leptin levels are low is the time when your set point can be changed. At this point, leptin is trying to find its way back to pre-pregnancy levels, both quantitatively and functionally. As it does so, it's open to suggestions from you. Like a computer, you can reprogram yourself. If you do the things that induce leptin levels to return too quickly, like eat lots of fat, you will not only gain weight, of course, but you will also reset your set point higher. If you allow leptin to seek its own level and return to full force gradually, according to nature's plan, you can lower your set point. Theoretically, your new set point weight is going to be reduced by the amount of weight you have lost up to now plus all the weight you will lose in the second weight loss trimester. Once your second or third normal period has arrived and your cycle of leptin, estrogen, and progesterone levels is secure, your set point is cemented and weight loss slows. As you already know, this will occur, in most cases, six months after delivery.

The trick, then, is to keep your leptin "happy" so that it does what it does best: diminish your appetite, burn fat, raise your metabolism, and oversee your monthly menstrual cycle. There are five ways to do this, and you already began doing some of them in the first weight loss trimester.

YOU CAN HELP YOUR FAT-BURNING HORMONE FIVE DIFFERENT WAYS!

1. Lower your total fat consumption.
2. Cut the fat at dinner.

3. Avoid eating after 8:00 P.M.

4. Take your vitamins.

5. Avoid foods that contain MSG.

Lower Your Total Fat Consumption

If you began the 30 percent fat eating style as outlined for the first weight loss trimester, you are already on your way to resetting your set point. Since leptin is the hormone of the fat cell, it responds to the amount of fat in your diet. The more fat you eat, the more fat you stuff into your fat cells. The more fat in your fat cells, the more active your fat cells become and the more leptin is made. The quicker the rise in leptin, the higher your set point, and the more difficult it becomes to lose weight. You want to lower your set point, not raise it. No one knows the exact amount of fat that you need to eat to lower your set point, but when you examine the food intakes of women who weigh less after delivery than before they were pregnant, most kept their daily fat intake between 25 and 30 percent total fat calories per day. Remember, each gram of fat contains 9 calories. A non-nursing mom consuming 1500 calories per day should limit her fat intake to about 500 calories (approximately 55 grams). For a nursing mom consuming 2000 calories per day (see Chapter Eight), 650 calories of fat (or 72 grams) should be the daily upper limit. To put this in perspective for you, a large order of french fries at McDonald's contains 320 calories, of which about 160 calories come from fat. That's really not that bad when you consider that Subway's cold-cut sub (one foot long) contains 853 calories, of which 360 are fat calories. The message to take home is: Learn the fat content and calorie counts of the foods you eat, so that you don't blow your whole day's fat quota on just one meal. Your leptin and your waistline won't like it!

Once again, let's introduce some common sense and a scale to this passion-filled discussion of *adipose* (fat) tissue.

Thousands of years ago, believe it or not, there were no cupcakes, ice cream, or Reese's peanut butter cups, and most of the fat that people ate came from the animal meats and dairy products that they consumed. The ancients revered fat. The Old Testament goes to great lengths in teaching us how to deal with the fat of sacrifices. Fat was considered a delicacy, worthy only of the priestly class! How things have changed — or have we become a nation of priests? A quick check of the number of fast-food restaurants and convenience stores in your neighborhood shows how far we have come. We have round-the-clock access to high-fat foods.

The 30-percent-fat figure that we are working with was established a few years ago when our national fat intake was approaching 45 percent. This high percentage was thought to contribute to the increasing incidence of blocked heart and brain arteries, either of which can kill people and both of which are common in industrialized countries where people eat lots of fat. Public health scientists wanted to lower our fat intake to 20 percent or less. Some experts even advocated a limit of 10 percent daily fat calories, with the idea that intake this low could actually reverse coronary artery disease.

Many of you may be surprised to learn that the average consumption of fat in this country has gone down over the past decade, while the amount of obesity has risen during this same time period. Does this make sense? It sure does when you look at the numbers a bit more closely. Average fat consumption has come down, all right, but not evenly across all weight groups. Desirable-weight women—Type A new moms, for example—have indeed cut back on their fat intake, while overweight and obese women (Type B and Type C, respectively) are probably eating higher fat-laden diets than ever before. This is a direct result of too many so-called "low-fat foods" being consumed in such high quantities. That's because we aren't able to avoid one fact of life: Fat tastes better, and we are creatures of taste and habit. *Taste rules!* Foods that are low in fat often taste like cardboard. A little less than 30 percent fat was found to be the lowest amount of daily fat intake that people could tolerate over time, while still enjoying the taste of their food and contributing to their good health, as well. Therefore, 30 percent is a compromise figure, but we'll take it! Again, *taste rules!* The ultimate decision about what goes into your mouth is based on the same criteria that will motivate your child to fight you tooth and nail in his or her high chair: No matter how nutritious the food, if it doesn't taste good, it's not going to be eaten.

Fat tastes *so* good! You can eat twenty low-fat cookies and still crave just *one* full-fat, or normal, cookie. You never see the opposite situation: No one finishes a cone of regular ice cream and says, "Wow, could I use some fat-free yogurt now!" If keeping your daily fat intake at 30 percent (or less) makes your leptin and your taste buds happy, do it!

The eating plan we suggest for the second weight loss trimester is an extension of the one you used in the first weight loss trimester. By now you should be well versed in the eating style behind the core menu plans. With continued practice, you will master the art of judging portions and nutrient content of all foods, especially fat-containing foods. Remember, you can always go back to the menu plans for guidance. Continually using the core menus as the template for your second trimester of weight loss will keep your postpartum leptin levels high for as long as possible, increasing your metabolism and fat-burning capabilities.

Complex carbohydrates help leptin, too. Recent research has revealed that leptin needs insulin to function better. Complex carbohydrates, as you know, encourage the release of insulin, which in turn will help leptin help you.

If you haven't already done so, try some of the recipes starting on page 217, which, by the way, are easy to prepare and, mercifully, *not* time-consuming.

There is one more thing that you should know about fat. Lately, there has been a great deal of attention paid in the media to so-called "good" fats and "bad" fats. Some new research has suggested that "bad" fats like the ones found in margarine clog the pipes of life, your coronary arteries, while the "good" fats found in such foods as butter are less likely to harm you. This story was picked up by the national media, who printed newspapers with headlines such as, "Butter is better for you than margarine."

Things have gotten out of hand. There really are no good or bad fats. Until we learn more about the effects of different types of fat on your body, play it smart. Limit your *total fat intake* to between one-quarter and one-third of your total daily food intake. If you think that you can't do it, then try this "can't miss" method of lowering your fat intake given to me by one of my patients who is a nurse. She told me to get some french fries from a local hamburger joint and put them in a blender. Next, add one to two cups of water and mix at high speed for one minute. Here is what you are left with: Since fatty oils float on water, the top of your blender will contain a thick, goopy, greasy film composed of the fat from the french fries. Underneath, you will see clear water! Just imagine this gooey mess clogging up your arteries. Try this experiment once, and you will never have to do it again. High fat is out!

To finish the second weight loss trimester with a bang, you need to fine-tune your fat intake in a way that keeps leptin in a good mood and helps pull your set point, and your weight, down.

Cut the Fat at Dinner

Many hormones, as part of your very own body clock, function on night-day cycles. Some rise in the evening, and some in the morning. These variances are thought to account for some well-known observations. The most common time for a woman to go into labor is 3:00 in the morning. Menstruation usually begins at 5:00 in the morning. You weigh the most at 6:00 in the evening, so never weigh yourself then! Both asthma attacks and spontaneous births peak at 4:00 in the morning. Speaking of spontaneous births, about ten babies are born each year in New York City cabs, and three on the subways! Four hundred babies are born each year in traffic jams in Bangkok, Thailand.

Your internal biological clock controls the timing of these hormonal peaks and valleys. Leptin is also on a timer. It rises at about 8:00 in the evening, peaks in the early morning hours, and then reaches its lowest level when most of us begin working. I call leptin the hormone of darkness. When you are sleeping or working the graveyard shift, your leptin comes out to play. Remember, leptin levels are responsive to fat, so you don't want lots of fat floating around in your blood. All this excess fat in your blood at night may confuse leptin, which is genetically programmed to operate in low-fat conditions. If your body senses that you have too much fat in your system at night, your brain sends a signal to your fat cells to lower the amount of leptin that your body makes. Less leptin means more of you, because low leptin levels slow your metabolism and increase your appetite. There are two ways to eat so as not to interfere with your natural leptin cycle. The first way is to be strict about limiting your fat intake to the 30-percent limit for the *evening* meal. This is a lot easier to do than you think. In fact, if you have been following the core menus, you are already doing it! Just *keep* doing it. After all, having complex carbohydrates like pasta along with low-fat protein sources such as fish and chicken for dinner is hardly suffering!

Remember, there are only a few weeks left until the six-month weight loss barrier descends. Leptin comes out at night to see how you are doing, and you need to put on a good show. You put on your best show when you limit your fat intake at dinner.

The second way to keep leptin on your side is by continuing to do something that you began in the first weight loss trimester.

Avoid Eating After Eight O'clock

In Chapter Six, we said that eating past 7:30 or 8:00 P.M. favors weight gain because that is when your metabolism slows. Now, we have another reason not to eat late. Eating late interferes with the message that leptin is trying to send your brain, a message of fullness and a directive to keep your metabolism up. Humans, like most mammals (unless they are nocturnal and sleep during the day), are genetically programmed not to eat when it gets dark. If you eat late, your body gets back at you by slowing your metabolism during the night, making it easier for fat to be deposited and, through a complicated process, increasing your food intake the following day. Therefore, you need a feeding time cutoff that will put you in sync with the rise in your leptin levels. Your weight loss success now depends on this simple lifestyle change: No eating at all past 8:00 P.M. That means no snippet of apple or celery, no sliver of cake, no low-fat cookie. Not even one potato chip, or that tiny handful of low-fat pretzels you are accustomed to enjoying. You may drink as much water or seltzer as you wish, but learn to finish eating before 8:00. Get up from the table, brush your teeth, and call it a night as far as eating is concerned. *Stay out of the kitchen.* Those of you who work late should eat at work and finish your meal prior to 8:00. Night-shift workers, beware: You will have a hard time losing weight if you eat at night. I have yet to see a night-shift worker lose weight and keep it off!

I tell all my patients who are trying to lose weight that the real secret of Hollywood stars is that they have trained themselves to go to sleep on an empty stomach. They know that eating big, fat-laden dinners is a recipe for disaster, or a shortcut to becoming sumo wrestlers. In Japan, sumo wrestlers are required to gain enormous amounts of weight to help them in their sport. They can weigh up to 500 pounds or more. To gain weight, sumo wrestlers drink beer and eat rice before they go to sleep! Keep in mind that alcohol, per gram, has almost the same amount of calories as fat, *so watch your alcohol intake too!*

No food after 8:00 P.M.! Let your body clock tick in your favor!

Take Your Vitamins

Your body is still in a repair mode and needs vital nutrients and vitamins. The restoration project your body began after delivery may take up to one year to complete. Maintain the vitamin intake that we specified for the first weight loss trimester. You should probably take your prenatal vitamin formulas and mineral supplements that we outlined in Chapter Six for at least nine months postpartum. After that you can switch to a more generalized product, with one caveat. Be certain that your vitamin supplement, along with the food that you eat, supplies at least 400 micrograms of the vitamin folic acid every day. Folic acid at this level can help prevent certain congenital malformations in a baby's central nervous system, should you become pregnant again. A new federal law mandates that folic acid must be added to enriched cereal and grain products such as flour, cornmeal, pasta, and rice. Breakfast cereals are required to be fortified with folic acid, too, which is great. However, not all cereals are created equal in the folic acid department. General Mills' Total and Kellogg's Product 19 are the best sources of folic acid among breakfast cereals. Keep in mind that you are getting plenty of folic acid by following the core menus because complex carbohydrates such as whole grain products, beans, and peas are excellent sources of folic acid. Folic acid is also found in protein sources such as fish, eggs, and milk.

New research has demonstrated that vitamins may play a role in how leptin works. In your brain, leptin interfaces with your neurotransmitters such as serotonin and noradrenalin. In Chapter Six, we learned that certain vitamins and minerals help neurotransmitters function at optimal levels. Among these are vitamin B_6 and the mineral zinc. It's not a far stretch to imagine that these same nutrients would help the performance of leptin, so be certain that your vitamin supplement contains sufficient amounts of zinc and B_6. The vitamin and mineral chart on page 85 lists the daily requirements for these important nutrients.

There are two other vitamins that you need to increase now. They are vitamins C and E. I call them *the* vitamins of the second trimester of weight loss. Both vitamin C and vitamin E are antioxidants. Antioxidants are substances that help cells function better. Each day of your life, your cells generate waste products, or *toxins*, that must be eliminated. Some of these toxins are called "free radicals," and some free radicals may be harmful to your body. Excess free radical formation has been implicated in premature aging and in certain cancers. Antioxidants such as vitamins C and E fight these toxins by keeping cell membranes strong and by helping the cells destroy toxins. I like to think of these two vitamins as cell stabilizers and scavengers. Weight loss involves the breakdown of fat cells. The cells don't literally break, but tiny holes are created in their outer walls, or membranes, through which microscopic fat droplets are released into the blood. Vitamin C keeps the fat cell membrane in top condition, and vitamin E helps scavenge any breakdown products that sneak out when fat leaves the fat cell. I recommend that all non-nursing new moms take 500 milligrams of vitamin C and 200 international units of vitamin E daily. Many of you may be tempted to increase your vitamin C and E intake even more. My advice: Don't! There is new research to suggest that at higher doses these antioxidants become pro-oxidants, which means that they *promote* the formation of toxins!

If you are nursing, consult your health professional before increasing your vitamin intake.

You should be aware that many soy-based complex carbohydrates, along with red grapes, romaine lettuce, and tomatoes, also contain antioxidants. That's because they contain beta-carotene, a powerful antioxidant similar to the one found in vitamin A. Nursing women should never increase their intake of vitamin A above the currently suggested level of 1300 micrograms per day. Vitamins get into breast milk, and since vitamin A is fat-soluble, it gets stored in the liver quite easily, where it can build to toxic levels and harm your baby and you. This condition is called "hypervitaminosis A." Symptoms include visual disturbances, loss of appetite, nausea, behavior problems, and cracking skin. If you notice any of these symptoms, stop whatever supplement you are taking and call your doctor.

Avoid Foods Containing MSG

There has been a new development regarding the food additive monosodium glutamate, or MSG. It appears as if MSG can actually block leptin from functioning properly. Incredibly, it seems that MSG may play a role in obesity. The best thing, then, is to avoid foods that contain MSG, including canned soups, some crackers, and packaged dry fruits. When you go to a Chinese restaurant, ask the waiter for MSG-free food. Be sure to read labels, especially those on processed foods, because many times MSG is hidden on the label under a mountain of food ingredients. Breast-feeding women should be on the lookout for any product containing MSG because it is transferred to a nursing infant. High levels of MSG can be toxic to an infant's nervous system, which is why it was removed from baby food.

TONE IT DOWN

Almost every new mom has certain areas that have bulged, spread, or fanned out during her pregnancy. These "problem areas" are the sites that took the brunt of your body changes and need some special attention. They include the thighs, hips, and buttocks. These areas can be toned and reshaped if you give it a try. I believe that it is best to attack this problem as soon as possible, but as you know from the first trimester of weight loss, some of you may have had medical procedures such as cesarean sections that prevented you from performing toning exercises. Or perhaps you were too tired or just weren't "into it." If you haven't started, now is the time. If you have started toning your muscles of the pelvic floor as outlined on page 90, that's great. Just be certain to check with your doctor before beginning any type of postpartum exercise plan.

Like the six-month weight loss barrier, I believe that there is a time frame that must be respected if you are going to redefine your body's contours. Every day in the gym, I see middle-aged women trying to shrink down the same problem areas they developed during long-ago pregnancies. Don't you think they wish that they could have started earlier, when their bodies were more elastic and malleable? You are now in that position! By doing some toning exercises in the postpartum, you can accomplish wonderful things that are unimaginable at any other time. Common sense tells you that it becomes harder to tone as the years go by, so do it now!

Remember, this is not about losing weight—it's about toning and sculpturing your muscles. Pregnancy is very tough on your muscles, tendons, ligaments, and support tissues. You have stretched yourself out over the past year; now, it's time to snap back. It's amazing how a few minutes per day doing proper toning movements can restore and reshape those parts of your body that your pregnancy altered. The *Hello, Baby! Good-bye, Baby Fat!* muscle toning and tightening plan was designed by Dr. Marks (whom you met in Chapter Six). The program is designed for all new moms, breast-feeding or not, no matter what your level of fitness is. If you are currently doing some other form of exercise that does not include toning movements, these are perfect for you! Dr. Marks has developed a simple, nontaxing program that gives the quickest results possible. You will even learn how to tone your abdomen *without* doing sit-ups.

Your job is to stay dedicated to your toning movements for a few minutes each day. Find a comfortable, well-ventilated spot in your house, wear loose-fitting clothes, start the music, and let's go! One rule to follow: Never hold your breath when performing any exercise; it puts too much stress on your heart, lungs, and other parts of your body. Move and breathe, breathe and move. Also, there should be plenty of water available in case you get thirsty. If you have a friend who has just delivered, or who just wants to get better tone, then work out together!

One word of caution: Lately many women's magazines and television spots have featured workouts that show new moms holding their infants while exercising. Some actually incorporate the baby into the workout, as if the child were a dumbbell! I strongly recommend that you do not do this. Your baby is no dumbbell! It is unfair, in my opinion, to put your baby in harm's way by making him or her part of your workout. Why risk injury to your baby and yourself? When you exercise, you should be focused on *your* body, not your baby's.

THE "3-T" TONE AND TIGHTEN PLAN

The *Hello, Baby! Good-bye, Baby Fat!* muscle toning and tightening plan is called the "3-T" plan because it contains three bonuses for you, and they all begin with the letter "T." They are:

1. **Time:** Your toning program will take only a few minutes a day.

2. **Target:** Your program targets those groups of muscles that have been hardest hit by your pregnancy, such as the thighs, hips, abdomen, and buttocks.

3. **Trim:** The best part about doing toning exercises now is that they can keep you trim years from now!

Chairwoman of the Board

A quick glance at the diagrams on the following pages shows that all of your toning exercises are to be performed using a chair. The chair is not a silent prop; it's important. The chair provides you with support and takes the strain off other parts of your body that are not involved in a particular movement. Keep in mind that your body has changed so much during your pregnancy that even your center of gravity is altered. Your balance, therefore—especially if you are overweight—is probably a bit off. The chair offers you comfort and stability. Think of it as your workout partner. The "3-T" plan is designed to use your legs (which in the postpartum are heavier than normal) as weights. Therefore there is no need for you to add any weights to these exercises.

In the end, what you put into your toning exercises will determine what you get out of them. The entire program can be done in as little as five to ten minutes a day, but don't do the program just to go through the motions. Do your toning movements with vigor and conviction! The new *toned* and *tightened* YOU will be your reward!

Another feature of the "3-T" plan is that these tightening and toning movements allow you to work on several problem areas at the same time because different muscle groups are working together to generate the movement. Let's get your toning program off the ground with some stomach work.

The "Tummy Tuck"

Do you like doing sit-ups? Do you know anyone who does? It's great to know that you don't have to do sit-ups to tighten your tummy. In fact, our first toning movement, the "tummy tuck," can be thought of as an "un-sit-up" because you never even leave your chair. There are three steps to the "tummy tuck": A, B, and C.

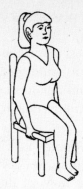

STEP A: Begin by grasping both sides of your chair and sitting straight up.

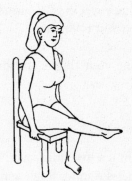

STEP B: Keeping your left leg planted on the floor, extend your right knee and raise it slightly off the chair.

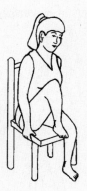

STEP C: Continuing the same motion, bend your right leg and bring it upward toward your chest (do your best). Once your leg is as close to your body as possible, tighten your stomach muscles, and hold for a five-second count. Slowly return your leg to the seat of the chair, relax, and breathe.

After you finish the right leg, repeat the same steps: A, B, and C, this time using your left leg. You should try and do between five and ten repetitions with each leg, and of course you can alternate sides with each repetition. If you feel strong enough, you can eventually try both legs at the same time!

We call this exercise the "tummy tuck" because of the way that you tuck your knee into your chest. Besides working the abdomen, the tummy tuck also works the front of the thigh and your shoulders because of the way that you are holding on to the chair. By the way, if you find that holding on to the seat of the chair is too hard, use a chair that has arms. After a few weeks your tummy will become trimmer and your posture will have improved, too.

Now it is time to tone your thighs and buttocks. To do this you will have to stand up!

The "Thigh Slammer"

This toning movement is a true time-saver, because it tones two problem areas at the same time: the inner thigh and the outer thigh. You should be aware that separate muscle groups control these areas. Working just the outer thigh, for instance, does nothing to tone the inner thigh. The "thigh slammer" tones both with one movement, so let's get up and try this one. The "thigh slammer" also consists of three steps: A, B, and C.

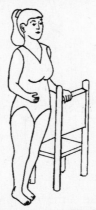

STEP A: Stand to the side, toward the back of your chair, as in the illustration.

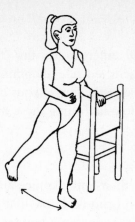

STEP B: Hold on to the back of your chair. Keep your right leg straight, and bring it out to your right side as far as you comfortably can. Hold this position for five seconds. Then relax and take a deep breath.

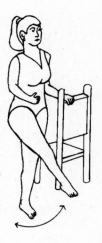

STEP C: As you bring your right leg back down, cross it in front of your left leg and continue to swing it over as far as you comfortably can. Hold this crossed-over position for five seconds, relax, and breathe.

Hold on to the chair with your other hand and repeat the same sequence, using your left leg. Do five to ten repetitions per day, minimum. You may notice one thing about the "thigh slammer" right away. First of all, you may not have the same flexibility and range of motion that you had before you were pregnant. Don't worry; it will all come to you as you lose weight! In any event, unless you are a gymnast or a ballet dancer, your leg will only be able to extend out two or three feet at most in Step B.

Besides your inner and outer thighs, the "thigh slammer" works other muscles including selected side abdominal muscles, called the *obliques*, and your buttocks. Speaking of your buttocks, the third toning movement is the key to establishing those dream buns.

The "Bun Burner"

Everyone, it seems, wants their buttocks nice and firm, and with good reason. Esthetics aside, you should know that the buttocks muscles, popularly known as buns, are very important for supporting your lower back and pelvis. Not only will toning movements get your buns into great shape, but they can also protect your lower back and spine from injury. Three quick steps and you have performed the "bun burner."

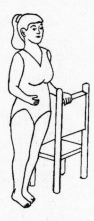

STEP A: Assume the same starting position as in the previous exercise.

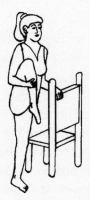

STEP B: Standing upright and tall, bend your right knee, and lift it as far up into your chest as you possibly can. At first you will only be able to get partially up. Hold the knee in this position for a count of five, let your leg down, relax, and breathe deeply.

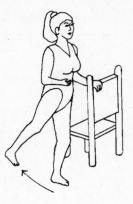

Now swing your bent leg back and upward as if you were trying to touch the back of your head! Nobody, unless they are a contortionist, can actually touch their head, so don't worry if you fall short; everyone does! When your leg is as far back as it can comfortably go, tighten your buttock muscles and hold for a five-second count. Then relax and take a nice deep breath.

Hold on to the chair with your other hand and repeat the same sequence, this time using your left leg. You should do five to ten repetitions for each leg. The "bun burner" exercise also works the thighs and, in particular, the back muscles of the thighs, or the hamstrings.

You see, I told you this would be easy. Just wait and see what you are going to look and feel like in a few weeks, tightened and toned!

The "Calf Hacker"

There is only one toning movement remaining. I call it the "calf hacker." The "calf hacker" is a variation of the common "toe raise" but with some added zest. It may help those of you who suffer from varicose veins.

During pregnancy, many women develop enlarged, engorged leg veins, known as varicose veins. This is thought to occur because of the tremendous pressure that the developing fetus puts on the blood flow in the lower extremities. Especially hard hit are the small valves that control blood flow in your veins, much as a lock controls water flow through a canal. If you can improve the pumping action inside the vein, you take pressure off the valve and improve blood flow, reducing varicose veins. The best way to propel blood through your leg veins, short of brisk running, is to use your calf muscles as a pump. A few minutes each day practicing the two steps of the "calf hacker," and you can begin to shrink those varicose veins down.

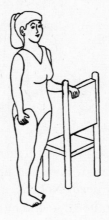

Begin using the same starting position as in Step A in the previous exercise, above.

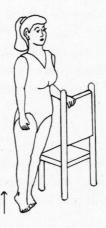

STEP A: Standing straight, with both feet together, rise up on tiptoes as high as you can go. Hold for a count of two and visualize squeezing your calf muscle. The next step is a downward return movement with a little flair.

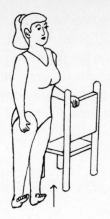

STEP B: With your feet still together, bring your feet slowly back down to the starting position. As soon as your heels touch the floor, lift the front of your feet off the floor and force your toes backward and up ("dorsiflex"), as if you want them to touch your shins. This last movement really stretches your calf muscles and your hamstrings, and it promotes blood flow up your legs and back to your heart. When you get used to doing the "calf hacker," you can do it anytime you are on your feet. For maximum benefit, I suggest doing twenty-five repetitions, two times a day.

THE ULTIMATE PERSONAL TRAINER

Despite how much these toning exercises can help, there are many women who just hate exercising and won't do it. Let me share with you the story of one woman who had a special angel helping her tone.

Wanda A., a 31-year-old telephone operator and devout Elvis fan, delivered twin boys. Wanda had gained 55 pounds during her pregnancy and was still 10 pounds overweight. More than anything, she needed a good toning program, because it seemed like her thighs had borne the brunt of her pregnancy, and they still showed it! But Wanda had never exercised in her life. Now, three months postpartum, she was no closer to breaking this pattern. One day, while going through her large collection of Elvis memorabilia, she noticed for the first time that she had unconsciously categorized her entire Elvis Presley collection according to the way Elvis looked. There was the "heavy Elvis" and the "thin Elvis." Suddenly it dawned on her that she didn't want to categorize her own life that way. To motivate herself to start moving, she put two pictures of Elvis on her wall. One was of a thin rock-and-roller being inducted into the Army, and the other was a later picture of her idol in a white sequined jumpsuit, obviously overweight. With Elvis looking down at her, she finally began to whip herself into shape. Wanda had found the ultimate personal trainer! What will it take to motivate *you?*

"HOW MUCH WEIGHT WILL I LOSE?"

I knew that sooner or later you were going to ask me that. I have seen *tremendous* weight loss by overweight new moms in the second trimester of weight loss. Even if you were to average just two pounds lost per week, after six months you would have lost . . . well, you know what that comes out to! That would be ideal for many of you, but in reality, your weight loss slows as you approach the six-month barrier, and most of your weight will be lost during the first part of the second trimester of weight loss. How much weight you lose is dependent on your sticking closely with the program and on your genetics. Any doctor who specializes in weight loss will tell you, though, that the weight loss efforts of Type B and Type C new moms are inspirational to us all, because they, like you, do so well!

WORKING, THE WEIGHT LOSS "TRUMP CARD"

During the first weight loss trimester, you spent a lot of energy getting the mind/body connection just right. As many of you return to work, there are some new issues to deal with. The emotional issues that surround leaving your new baby have, naturally, already surfaced. Guilt and worry must be balanced against financial and practical considerations. These include making the proper child care arrangements and planning to pump breast milk at work, if you choose to do so. Nearly 70 percent of women of childbearing age are in the workforce. This means that each year almost three million postpartum women have to come grips with making the transition from home to workplace. Many of you will find yourselves wearing two new hats: one as a first-time mother, and the other as a new working mother. I hope things work out for you. (Excuse the pun!) There is a third hat that postpartum women wear, too: that of weight loss champion!

One of the surprising discoveries about postpartum weight loss is that women who return to work earliest lose more weight and lose it faster than women who stay home. An even more incredible finding was that working women, even without exercising, lost more weight then those women who stayed home and did exercises! Somehow, going to work opened up a whole new arena for weight loss!

Why should this be? Is it just a question of vanity and the need to survive in a competitive business world? Perhaps some of you are thinking that working women fare better because they are not at home, exposed to food 24 hours a day. There is some support for this idea because women who work at home do not lose as much weight as women who work outside the home. However, if this were the sole reason for the disparity, you would only find overweight women at home and only thin new moms at work, and we all know that this is not the case.

One piece of the puzzle was furnished by a study that showed that women who worked outside the home on a volunteer basis did not lose as much weight as those women who had paying jobs. Was it the money, then, I wondered? Or was it a function of the type of work that a woman does? It turns out that it makes no difference what type of work a new mom does; she will still lose more weight than her stay-at-home counterparts. Blue collar, white collar, no collar, it makes no difference. I still was no closer to understanding what was going on.

Then one day, three generations of the Lane family walked into my office on a weight loss mission. They made me understand! Hailing from Adamstown, in beautiful Lancaster County, Pennsylvania, there was C. J., the youngest (age 20) and 30 pounds overweight, with most of it residing on her hips and thighs. Her mother Carolyn (age 42) was about 40 pounds overweight. The matriarch, Grandma Lucy (age 60), could stand to lose 30 pounds herself. I saw them once in consultation, and since my office was a five-hour drive from their hometown, I told them we could schedule appointments every three months, rather than the usual two-week visits that are the normal practice. I never heard from them again.

One year later, an envelope arrived full of wedding photos. The

Lanes had neglected to tell me that the reason they all wanted to lose weight was C. J.'s upcoming wedding. The photos were of svelte Lucy, Carolyn, and C. J. having a ball at the wedding. There was no card, no inscription, nothing but pictures. I understood what had happened. It was something that went beyond the dry facts of weight loss, and something that I have seen before. Women who try to lose weight for an upcoming wedding almost always succeed! They may not all walk down the aisle as thin as runway models, but they nearly always lose substantial amounts of weight, requiring about sixty dress fittings! The need to be thinner in front of a crowd is a tremendous impetus for weight loss: If a woman has just discovered that she has diabetes or high blood pressure and is told to lose even a few pounds for reasons of health, she may not do as well as the woman who wants to lose weight for an upcoming wedding.

What does this have to do with weight loss and a return to work? Plenty! It shows that, genetics and hormones aside, the human mind can rise above any biologically imposed weight disadvantage. There are certain times when *what* and *how much* you put into your mouth is controlled not by hunger but by a conscious mind making smarter weight loss choices. Weddings are one of these times, and so is a return to work after pregnancy.

GREAT WEIGHT LOSS MINDS THINK ALIKE

The pressure on women to regain their former shape in a competitive workplace is enormous. Working women try to fit into their old work clothes and working minds as soon as possible after delivery. Most often, they succeed. The lesson to be learned here is *not* for the working mother; it's for the non-working new mom. She is at risk of losing less weight than a working mom, all things being equal. What the Lane family and working women really teach us is that proper *focus* combined with a realistic goal can take you a long way. These are intangibles that aren't easily explained, but I'll try.

I believe that the weight loss success of the Lane family and of women returning to work is predicated on their using a part of the brain that is higher than the appetite control center, both anatomically and functionally. It is called the *cerebral cortex*. It's also known as a "higher" brain center, and it contains much of the essence of who you are, including your sense of self, your memories, your creative powers, and your reasoning abilities. In addition, it's the abode of your spirituality. The higher center of your brain is also your food boss, because the ultimate decision about what you put into your mouth must first be cleared by the cerebral cortex. For instance, many religions require fasts: consider Ramadan for Muslims and the Day of Atonement for Jews. On these special occasions, biology takes a backseat to religion, and even the most food-obsessed individual is able to voluntarily curb his or her appetite. The same dynamics operate during political-protest fasts. Even though food is all around you, you, too, can voluntarily raise your tolerance to cutbacks in your food intake, *if the stakes are high enough!* Weddings increase the stakes, and so does a return to work. It becomes a goal-oriented, spiritual type of weight loss.

This is not the same thing as willpower. Willpower almost always denotes a negative, self-denial approach. Your internal dialogue with yourself sounds like this, repeated over and over: "I want to eat this but I won't, because if I eat it, I will get fat, hate myself even more, and then eat lots more." This is usually a self-fulfilling prophecy and helps explain why you can't just will away a weight problem. You can't just wake up on January 2 with a New Year's resolution to lose weight and succeed in doing so.

I believe that there is even a biological difference between using willpower for weight loss and the more goal-oriented approach leading to weight loss. More than likely, different neurotransmitters are involved, creating cerebral-emotional responses that can range from the self-denying negativity of dieting and willpower to the inspired, almost transcendent, efforts involved in religious and political fasts. To be successful you must choose the right mind-set, the one that will reinforce the activity of your higher brain center.

The Lanes and women who return to work teach us that the mind can cultivate a more positive, enabling way to exert control. Sometimes, you just need an external push to get you there. This push can come from religion or from your political beliefs. But it can also come from your wanting to get thinner for a family get-together or your return to the workplace. In all of these situations, you have to answer to a higher authority than willpower: yourself!

The message for stay-at-home moms is that it just may be that remaining in the house makes it a little too easy not to go for that goal-oriented weight loss approach. You need a change of scenery. You need to cultivate activities outside of the house, activities that exercise your mind and your body. I can't tell you how many women who have just delivered told me that for various reasons they tended to remain at home for the first few months after delivery. One woman told me that the only exercise she got for the first few postpartum months was to get the mail! These new moms remained in isolation. Of course, this type of behavior could be a result of postpartum depression. However, working new moms, depressed or not, are still more successful at weight loss than those moms who stay at home. Leaving the house, then, must in itself have some sort of emotional significance that involves your brain's neurotransmitters. One that comes to mind immediately is that when you feel good about yourself, you raise your levels of endorphins, which make you feel even better! A great way to start off the endorphin-raising process is by going for walks. You already know that exercise has no effect on postpartum weight loss, but getting out of the house and walking should not be looked upon as exercise for your body, but as exercise for your mind. A daily walk of fifteen minutes or more, done for YOUR sake, can furnish the same mind-set that working women achieve when they leave the house. Perhaps it's an internal symbol of exerting your independence. Remember, women who worked at home did no better at losing weight than women who stayed home and did not work. The idea, then, is this: Get a life outside the house. For the first few months, you may have needed to stay close to the house; now it's time for a change. Get dressed up. Go out and do things like visit friends, meet for lunch, find a new hobby, garden, visit museums, go to the movies, go to parks, and take leisurely car rides. Visit your house of worship. Most of these activities can be done with baby in tow. Just have fun! And heed the voice in the movie *Poltergeist* that said, "Get out!"

THE SIX MONTHS ARE UP!

For many of you Type B moms, and some Type C moms, the time has come. You certainly have accomplished a lot, but could the six-month weight loss barrier have arrived so quickly? I guess it has. With a little luck, one day we will figure out why this wall of time blocks further postpartum weight loss. In any event, I hope that you enjoyed yourself these past one hundred and eighty days, and that your baby is doing well. In a few short months it will be his or her first birthday.

I also hope that you have acquired and practiced the skills to help you keep the weight off now that your body chemistry has reverted to its pre-pregnancy state. If you aren't nursing, be sure to read the Epilogue, "The Future of Weight Loss," and find out how to maintain your new body in the years ahead.

Chapter Eight

Six to Nine Months Postpartum: The Third Trimester of Weight Loss

The final weight loss trimester begins and ends with breast-feeding. You already know that if you nurse, you should begin right at birth, and since you already know that six months postpartum is when weight loss screeches to a halt, how can we still be talking about breast-feeding and weight loss now? It's simple, really: Only certain women who breast-feed six months or longer will lose weight in the third trimester.

Just when it seems that your body has exhausted all of its weight loss tricks, it surprises you. A unique hormonal mechanism makes it possible for some nursing moms to get one last shot at smashing through the six-month weight loss barrier and continue to get thinner.

Who are these nursing moms who defy time? If the statistics are right, desirable-weight Type A moms reap no weight loss benefit from nursing and actually risk weight gain. The new moms who benefit the most from long-term breast-feeding are the women that need it the most: overweight Type B new moms or obese Type C new moms, age 30 and over. If this is you, you are very lucky.

BREAST-FEEDING: WEIGHT LOSS FROM THE HEART

After years of declining interest in long-term nursing on the part of new moms, the latest position paper on this subject from the American Academy of Pediatrics is bound to shake things up. In a new set of breast-feeding guidelines released at the end of 1997, the Academy strongly urges that infants be breast-fed exclusively with mothers' milk for at least the first year of life and for as long as mutually desirable thereafter. Now, that's radical! They didn't waver or compromise. Their recommendations are clear. To glean all of breast-feeding's health benefits, you must nurse for ONE YEAR! Are you prepared for that?

What's behind these new recommendations? They are based on the conclusions of a task force of health professionals who examined data gathered from developed nations in the Americas and Europe. The task force found that breast-fed babies seemed to have far fewer medical problems than formula-fed babies. Currently, only 50 percent of new moms nurse, and most for only a few weeks. Furthermore, many combine breast milk with formula.

The task force also offered some interesting suggestions that you should know about. They believe that babies should be breast-fed during the first hour after delivery, and that breast-fed babies should receive no water, sugar solutions, or formula unless medically indicated. In addition, the task force recommended that babies should be fed whenever they show signs of hunger, which include increased movements of the mouth, increased general activity, and alertness. They say you should not wait until your baby cries before you nurse. Crying is considered a late-stage indicator of hunger wherein the baby is already frust ted and uncomfortable.

The health enefits of nursing cited by the task force benefit both baby and mom, and are listed below. They are compiled from an article, "Breastfeeding and the Use of Human Milk," published in the December 1997 issue of the journal *Pediatrics*. You can review it yourself in the library, find it on the Internet, or ask your health care provider for a copy.

The Best of Health from Breast-Feeding, for Baby

The benefits of breast-feeding to baby are:

1. **Fewer Childhood Infections:** Breast-fed babies have fewer and less severe ear infections, less diarrhea, fewer urinary tract infections, and a lower incidence of serious medical disorders such as meningitis and pneumonia.

2. **Protection Against Certain Serious Medical Problems:** It is believed by many doctors that breast-feeding may help protect a baby against sudden infant death syndrome (SIDS), lymphoma, insulin-dependent diabetes, allergies, Crohn's disease and ulcerative colitis. The latter two are serious diseases that involve the gastrointestinal tract.

3. **Improved Teeth:** Breast-fed children have better teeth because factors in breast milk seem to prevent tooth decay. Babies who are nursed also get fewer cavities than formula-fed babies due to the higher sugar content of formula.

4. **Increased Cognitive Skills:** Breast-fed children may develop parts of their brain that allow them to do better on standardized tests.

5. **Better General Health:** Breast-fed children may be healthier overall. They are three times less likely to be hospitalized than bottle-fed babies.

6. **Less Risk of Obesity as Adults:** Babies who are nursed may have a decreased incidence of becoming overweight as adults.

The Best of Health from Breast-Feeding, for Mom

The benefits of breast-feeding to Mom:

1. **Immediate Health Benefits:** Moms who breast-feed have less postpartum bleeding, a more rapid return to normal uterine size, and less menstrual blood loss during the postpartum period.

2. **Later Health Benefits:** Moms who breast-feed reduce their risk for hip fractures, ovarian and premenopausal breast cancer, and, perhaps, uterine cancer.

You will probably take all of these potential health benefits into consideration when you decide to breast-feed and for how long. Keep in mind, however, that breast-feeding does not guarantee health for you or your baby. The two lists above are based on statistical evidence, which means that breast-fed babies and their moms are more LIKELY to garner health benefits than those moms and babies are who not involved in nursing.

Are you breast-feeding? How long do you plan to continue? Right now, only one out of every five new moms breast-feeds beyond six months, and most of them are combining breast-feedings with formula. The number of women who breast-feed their infants has declined by 20 percent since the 1930s, when almost 70 percent of women breast-fed. It remains to be seen whether a pro-nursing trend will emerge after the new guidelines are put into practice.

One presumed health benefit is missing from this list of mom's benefits. I omitted this benefit on purpose: weight loss! The authors of the study claim, "Recent research demonstrates that lactating women have an earlier return to pre-pregnant weight." I disagree, and strongly.

NURSING: TREASURE CHEST OF WEIGHT LOSS?

The relationship between weight loss and breast-feeding is one of the most misunderstood areas of the postpartum experience, and we are going to clear it up right now. We had better, because before you commit one year to breast-feeding, you should know all the facts. Obviously, no woman decides to nurse solely to lose weight, but what if you found out that breast-feeding actually causes weight gain? Wouldn't that be a factor in your ultimate decision to breast-feed? It should!

Yes, I know that your sister-in-law lost 45 pounds while breast-feeding, and that your doctor promised you would lose at least 10 pounds. Every mother has a breast-feeding weight loss story to tell. In fact, there are two million breast-feeding weight loss stories every year! I would like to share one of them with you.

One night, I had a magical experience. Unable to sleep in the wee hours of a summer night, I tiptoed downstairs to find my wife, Janette, nursing our infant daughter Alison. They were sitting by an open window in the dark, but their faces were lit by a full moon. They couldn't see me, but I could see the way that Janette was smiling at Alison, adoring the nursing baby, as they rocked slowly in contented silence. I realized that I was witnessing a living sculpture cast in lunar white. At that moment, I was viewing one of nature's most powerful bonds at work, the bond that exists between a mother and her nursing child.

I never told my wife that I was watching. Men, after all, can only be observers of a breast-feeding encounter, but what I saw turned me into an instant proponent of nursing.

It is interesting to note that a newborn's vision only extends about one foot. It must be comforting for the hungry baby to see its mother's face. I think that we have become far too scientific in our approach to breast-feeding. After all, women have been nursing naturally and instinctively for thousands of years. In fact, physical health considerations aside, possibly the best reason to breast-feed in the first place is to foster the mother-child bond.

Yes, breast-feeding's rewards are many; but, unfortunately, weight loss is not one of these rewards, unless you are an overweight mom who nurses for at least six months. This is the one area where old wives' tales continue to prevail, so let's get to the truth.

A review of the worldwide literature about breast-feeding and weight loss demonstrates a true weight loss inequality. Breast-feeding has essentially no effect on weight loss for younger, desirable-weight, first-time moms. Disturbingly, there are many carefully done studies that demonstrate that nursing not only caused some women to *gain* weight but that these women only lost weight when they stopped breast-feeding.

This is exactly what happened to Lisa Z., a 28-year-old accountant and second-time mom. Lisa did not breast-feed her first son because she had to return to work a few weeks after delivery, and she never mastered the logistical issues of breast-feeding and working full-time. Lisa followed a high complex carbohydrate and low-fat eating program and was back to her pre-pregnancy weight within three months.

After her second child was born, Lisa decided to stay home and breast-feed for as long as possible. She weighed 145 pounds at conception and gained 35 pounds with this pregnancy. Lisa began breast-feeding in the hospital, and by her six-week checkup she had lost 12 pounds. She was mystified when, within the next three weeks, and without changing any aspect of her food intake, she gained 6 pounds. The following month she gained another 8 pounds! Concerned, she notified her doctor, who told her that it was probably just her hormones readjusting to breast-feeding and that a small weight gain was really not that unusual. He made it sound like it was no big deal, but it was! Lisa continued to gain weight.

Due to a change in plans, Lisa had to return to work sooner than expected. She decided to stop breast-feeding on her first day back at the office. She weighed 168 pounds, 23 more than when she became pregnant. She joined Weight Watchers and managed to lose 10 pounds, but at the six-month barrier, Lisa's weight loss career ended, and her weight gain career began. Today, one year later, she weighs 160 pounds, 15 more than at conception! If she decides to have another child and gains her usual 35 pounds, she will risk weighing close to 200 pounds!

After all you have heard about breast-feeding's virtues, is this scenario even logical? It sure is. In fact, it's *bio-logical!*

MILK POWER

The notion that weight loss is caused by breast-feeding comes from the fact that nursing women burn extra calories making, storing, and expressing milk. You never know when your little one wants to eat, so a breast-feeding mom's body works overtime, 24 hours a day, to make milk. Whether you are watching T.V., sleeping, or reading a book, if you are nursing, you constantly produce breast milk. You don't actually feel anything, but inside there is plenty going on. The average nursing mom produces 23 ounces (750 milliliters) of milk per day. This production requires a plethora of hormonally induced biochemical "milk-making" activities that take place not only in the breast but in other parts of the body as well. All this activity burns calories!

Mother's milk contains nutrients derived from your body and from your diet. Among these nutrients is fat, of course, which your baby requires for its own growth and development. Like a new computer, your body comes preprogrammed to use your dietary fat before your body fat when forming breast milk. This is nature's guard against times of famine. When the food supply is scant, your body switches gears and utilizes your stores of body fat. Lest you think that famines existed only in biblical times, remember that much of Europe, from Ireland to Greece, has endured famine during this century. Today, with millions of people living under starvation conditions worldwide, one can go as far as Africa or as close as Appalachia to see how important a woman's fat-leaching capability is for human survival. This multifaceted mechanism is also what helps overweight nursing women lose weight in times of plenty!

How many calories per day do you burn making milk? In 1985, the World Health Organization put this figure at 750 calories per day, while many scientists claim it's closer to 650 calories per day. Remember, these numbers are estimates and your number can be different. Between 150 and 250 calories of this estimated 750-calorie total, or up to one-third, are derived from your body fat. The rest (about 500 calories) comes from your diet. This relationship, as we said, twists 180 degrees in times of starvation, when almost all of the fat in breast milk comes from the mother's body. Based on these numbers, it was decided that if the average nursing mom eats an extra 500 calories per day, she will provide enough calories for herself and her baby, and still lose weight. That's because if you subtract those 500 calories from the 750 calories you expend to make milk, you get a deficit of 250 calories per day. The implication is that even by increasing your food intake by up to 500 calories per day, you will still lose weight because breast-feeding and other activities use up all the extra calories and then some.

Remember, you need to eat 500 extra calories per day for each baby you nurse. If you have twins, you need an extra 1000 calories per day; with triplets it's an extra 1500 calories every single day!

The 500-calorie number is thrown around quite a bit by doctors, nurses, and nutritionists. In fact, the number "500" pops up in an obstetrician's office almost as often as the "Indianapolis 500" is mentioned in Indiana on Memorial Day weekend.

Five hundred calories is a lot of calories! World-class gymnasts may burn 500 calories during an hour-and-a-half workout. Sylvester Stallone, even during his most arduous *Rocky* workouts, would be lucky to burn 500 calories. Is your 500 calorie scheme even in the realm of common sense?

PROLACTIN POWER

There is yet another side to the breast-feeding and weight loss story that you should know about. It's the one that health care professionals don't like to discuss when touting the virtues of breast-feeding. Yes, you certainly burn a few hundred extra calories per day while your body prepares, stores, and secretes breast milk. But even with nature's gift of a free 24-hour workout, you still have no weight loss guarantee, because the same hormone that causes your milk to flow also *increases your appetite*.

This is a beautiful design by nature, once again showing off her sense of balance. Nursing moms need more food than at any other time in their lives, including pregnancy. It is ideal, then, to have the same hormone responsible for milk production also be the one to increase your appetite, allowing you to ingest enough calories to keep your milk factory up and running all day. This hormone is called *prolactin* (from the Latin *pro*, meaning "for"; and *lactin*, meaning "milk").

Prolactin is made in the pituitary gland in your brain and is involved in all facets of milk production. During pregnancy, prolactin rises to ten times its normal level and, along with estrogen and progesterone, causes your breasts to enlarge. Nature assumes that all women will breast-feed; hence all pregnant women get the increase in breast size.

If you decide not to nurse, a week or two after delivery, prolactin levels fall and your breasts return to normal size. If you nurse, your prolactin levels remain elevated, which keeps your breasts ready and able to supply all the nourishment that your newborn needs.

Each time your baby sucks on your nipple, your brain releases prolactin via a complex reflex involving nerve endings that connect the brain to the breast. The more intense the sucking action, the more prolactin is made and the more milk you produce. This is another shining example of the mind/body connection in action. In fact, the suction on your nipple also causes your uterus to contract, which helps you regain your figure. However, prolactin, like many other hormones we have confronted over the past six months, is two-faced.

Prolactin negates any weight loss calories that you expend making breast milk each day by making you want to eat more. If you breast-feed, no matter what you weigh, you will need more calories than at any other time in your life. Prolactin makes sure that you get them.

In a way that is not yet well understood, prolactin interfaces with serotonin and dopamine, along with other neurotransmitters, to increase your appetite. Some research suggests that prolactin may make you hungrier for high-fat foods like cheeses and peanuts. In any event, prolactin can make you hungrier than the entire 1998 Olympic champion U.S. women's hockey team after a tough game. You don't feel any different inside; you just eat. Again, this is just nature's way of ensuring that you have enough food to continue breast-feeding.

In a 1991 study, "Does Infant Feeding Method Influence Postpartum Weight Loss?" by Dr. S. Potter et al., published in the *Journal of the American Dietetic Association*, it was found that women who breast-feed lose less weight six weeks postpartum than women who formula-feed do. Although reasons cited for this observation include that breast-feeding women retain more fluids and have larger breasts, these results surprised even the authors. This same study also found no difference in weight loss at twelve months postpartum between desirable-weight women who nurse and those who do not.

It seems that you are caught up in one big biological "Catch-22." Nursing, the very process that burns calories and makes you thinner, can also make you heavier by causing you to eat more.

DRAWING A "MILK LINE" IN THE SAND

At about four to six months postpartum, a sudden, remarkable turn of events occurs that favors weight loss. Your milk hormone, prolactin, drops to its normal level *even if you are breast-feeding*. When prolactin falls, so does your appetite. You finally become a calorie-burning, breast-feeding weight loss machine with no strings attached.

This rather abrupt fall in prolactin levels is what allows the overweight and obese new mom to smash through the six-month weight loss barrier and continue to lose weight. Thinner moms do not fare as well and in general do not lose weight at this point. This may be due to the fact that thinner moms make less prolactin to begin with, and its fall at the four- to six-month mark is not as steep as the prolactin fall of overweight new moms. This difference in prolactin gradient may be the key, then, to women's weight loss while breast-feeding.

Weight loss at this point continues because you still are burning a few hundred calories a day making milk, although not as many as before, because your milk production slows over time. However, if you are careful about your food intake, you can continue to slim down for up to nine months, and sometimes even up to one year postpartum!

I call the six-month mark the "milk line" because, thanks to the departure of prolactin, this is where the health benefits of nursing and weight loss converge for an overweight nursing mom. Desirable-weight women who continue to breast-feed for the year-long period (or more) presumably get the health benefits without the weight loss.

For the overweight nursing mom, your old friend from the second weight loss trimester, leptin (the fat-melting hormone), returns to play a role in your newfound fat-burning ability. We know that the heavier you are, the more leptin your body makes, and pregnant overweight women make lots of leptin! We also know that there are connections between prolactin and leptin, since receptors for leptin are present in the breast and the area of the brain where prolactin is made. In addition, nursing postpones the return of a woman's period, and the signal to restart it most likely comes from leptin. As you know, leptin levels fall after delivery, and only when they rise to a high enough level can you have a period again. The exact relationship between nursing and your leptin levels is unclear at this time, but this much is certain: It is only with leptin's "permission" that your milk-making apparatus overrides your body's six-month weight loss clock.

And you always thought that thinner women had the weight loss advantage. Well, now you have one of your own.

GUILTY, OR NOT GUILTY? YOU DECIDE

You have your own reasons for choosing to breast-feed or not. Above all, breast-feeding should be an enjoyable experience for both you and your infant, a fact that sometimes seems to get lost when we scrutinize nursing so closely. The suggestions we make here are precisely that: suggestions. *You* are the boss. You decide the best course for you and your baby. If you decided not to breast-feed, don't feel guilty about your choice. If you were breast-feeding and found that a medical complication arose, or that it wasn't practical and didn't fit your lifestyle, you can still be the greatest mother in the world. After all, my mom was, and she didn't breast-feed.

There is absolutely no need to feel that you are withholding potential health benefits from your newborn by not breast-feeding. While many of the purported health benefits of breast-feeding are well documented, they are still statistical, not guarantees. You may breast-feed for two years and your child still may develop food allergies or asthma, or have frequent ear infections. Meanwhile, your bottle-feeding next-door neighbor may have kids who haven't been sick in years.

If you have any questions or concerns about breast-feeding, ask your health care practitioner. He or she may refer you to the local chapter of the La Leche League, an organization that champions breast-feeding. The La Leche League can provide you with a great deal of the latest literature or may refer you to a certified lactation specialist who has special training and expertise in the area of breast-feeding.

THE JOYS OF BREAST-FEEDING: MORE FOOD FOR YOU!

If you are an overweight new mom, it's easy to reconcile the joys of breast-feeding with the joys of weight loss. Breast-feeding and being overweight are a perfect match. You combine a woman trying to lose lots of excess weight with a process that burns lots of calories. Weight loss during nursing is an unexplored area in the medical literature, so many of you are weight loss pioneers. Your weight loss payoff is this: The third weight loss trimester may be the only time in your life when you can increase your food intake and still lose weight!

Your biggest stumbling block may be listening to your own doctor's advice. For years, doctors and nutritionists have recommended that a breast-feeding women consume 2700 calories per day, no matter what her initial weight was. This number was reached by adding the ubiquitous extra 500 calories to the average daily intake of 2200 calories recommended during pregnancy. The major concern was to make sure that breast-feeding women had enough food for their infants immediately after delivery. Unlike during pregnancy, when you were able to gain weight slowly because your baby needed time to grow, your new baby needs lots of food and now. Also, there was a concern that a woman wouldn't get enough vitamins and minerals from the typical American diet, something easily dealt with these days by taking supplements.

Let me tell you right now that the surest way for a nursing mom to sabotage her own weight loss success is to eat a diet close to 2700 calories a day, especially if she plans to nurse for a few months or more. Unless you are a world-class athlete, this is way too much food for you. You will do a lot better eating between 1800 and 2000 calories a day. This 1800-to-2000-calorie range is derived from an extensive review of the literature and, in particular, from a 1994 article entitled, "Effects of Dieting and Physical Activity on Pregnancy and Lactation" by Kathryn G. Dewey and Megan A. McCrory, published in the *American Journal of Clinical Nutrition*. This excellent review article helps answer questions regarding the safety of nursing and losing weight as well as exercising while nursing, which we will discuss shortly. The authors suggest that nursing women should not consume less than 1800 calories a day.

However, before we fix ideal daily calorie counts, let's deal with the issue of whether losing weight while nursing is safe. After all, you don't want to compromise the sole means of nourishment for your baby! These points sum up this important review article. They provide basic guidelines to new moms who want to balance nursing and weight loss.

• Rapid weight loss—that is, losing more than one pound per week after the first postpartum month—is not recommended. You already know that rapid weight loss leads to later weight gain, so why make this mistake?

• Breast-feeding moms should never limit the frequency or the duration of their feedings. This is extremely important. It's another way of saying, Don't withhold food from your baby because you are worried about your figure.

• Never go on a low-calorie diet while breast-feeding. Milk production in the first few weeks of nursing is often less then perfect in terms of both quality and quantity. It is during this time, right after birth, that women are often tempted to try low-calorie diets. Again, there is no need.

• Be sure to supplement your food intake with vitamins and minerals—but you already knew that!

• The numbers we have been discussing are for nursing single babies. That means you can eat up to 4000 calories a day for twins, and 6000 calories a day while nursing triplets. All mothers who nurse multiple babies should be under the guidance of a qualified nutritionist. The core menus contained in *Hello, Baby! Good-bye, Baby Fat!* do not provide adequate nutrients or calories for twins or triplets.

The core menus that you have been following since the first weight loss trimester contain daily suggestions for breast-feeding moms to provide both the extra calories and the protein content that they need. Calorie counts are extremely important now to ensure that you and your baby get adequate nutrition, especially considering that all of your baby's nourishment comes from one source only, your milk.

The core menus average 1650 calories per day. The added 500-calorie allowance for breast-feeders lifts the daily totals slightly above the 2000 calories per day that would lead to guaranteed weight loss. Nursing moms also need an extra 12 to 15 grams of protein per day, which can easily be achieved by eating two egg whites, two teaspoons of peanut butter, or one cup of yogurt, for example. These extra protein requirements are also included in the menu plans. To weigh less than you weighed before you were pregnant, use these menus as a template for honing your skills at following the complex carbohydrate/moderate fat system, because nursing moms are not immune to the effects of postpartum depression. Nursing moms are also subject to the whims of their fat-burning hormone, leptin, that influence the second weight loss trimester. Remember, having a free pass to consume an extra 500 calories must not be taken lightly. Nursing, like pregnancy, should not be looked upon as an excuse to eat for two. Moreover, filling up your extra quota of 500 calories per day with junk food does nothing for your baby and nothing for you, except make you heavier and unhealthy.

30 PERCENT FAT RULES!

If there was ever a time to limit your fat intake to 30 percent of your daily caloric totals, it is now. Common sense tells us why.

Your breast-feeding body now has a 24-hour need for fat as an energy source to foster milk production. As we noted above, your body preferentially utilizes the fat from your food as opposed to using your own body stores of fat. If you limit the amount of fat in your diet, you trick your body into thinking that you are living under starvation conditions. When this occurs, your body automatically starts chipping away at your fat reserves for the energy it needs to make milk.

It has not been determined how low-fat you should go, because we lack long-term studies on fat consumption in nursing mothers. You and your baby need a certain amount of fat for proper body functioning. There is one study of African women whose diets consisted of a mere 15 percent fat while nursing. When their breast milk was analyzed, it was found to contain adequate amounts of fat for proper growth. Until more research is done, however, I think that it is wise to stick to the format that you began months ago: 30 percent fat calories. Thirty percent fat makes your food taste good (and your breast milk, too!), provides enough essential fats for your baby's growth, and helps your weight loss as well.

As an added bonus, nursing women who limit their fat intake have been found not only to *increase* their milk production, but also to secrete milk that has a higher protein content!

NURSING: MOVING AND LOSING

Breast-feeding, exercise, and weight loss, anyone? The unique biochemical makeup of an overweight woman who breast-feeds allows for one great exception to the concept that exercise plays little role after delivery. Experience has shown that for many overweight and obese new moms, exercise may hasten and increase weight loss. Strange as it may seem, the entire issue of exercise and nursing is virtually unexplored in the medical literature, so it's back to our common sense once more. Unless you have a medical condition that would make exercising inadvisable, there is no reason not to exercise, and one great reason to exercise.

We've noted that nursing women are exercising internally, burning calories by making milk 24 hours a day. The process of milk production raises your metabolism. If you add a bit of daily exercise that further raises your metabolism, you get a synergistic or additive effect on your calorie burning and weight loss. Let's not forget that we are in the third weight loss trimester, when weight loss has stopped for most other postpartum women. To have an advantage like this right now is a wonderful thing. The type of exercise you do is unimportant. Try to find a form of exercise that will allow you to spend time outdoors and that you will enjoy, such as walking. By the way, the muscle toning and tightening plan of the second weight loss trimester is great for nursing new moms too! Just make certain that you obtain medical clearance before beginning any postpartum exercise program.

Some of you may be concerned about the effects of exercise on your breast milk. In the past, doctors have been somewhat "down" on the idea of nursing women exercising. They were worried that exercise might diminish the amount of milk produced or would increase its acidity, making it less tasty to the baby, who, in turn, would drink less. Two large review articles examined this issue and reached two conclusions:

- Exercise does not diminish milk production.
- Moderate exercise does not alter the taste of milk, and there is no evidence to date that babies of exercising moms drink less milk.

Exercise in the third trimester of weight loss for overweight and obese new moms is an ideal "win-win" situation; you enjoy all of the benefits of exercise and, unlike thinner new moms, you lose weight!

SPECIAL NURSING CONCERNS

You deserve the chance to breast-feed for as long as you want. Unfortunately, larger women have more problems with breast-feeding than their thinner counterparts. Thinner women often cite a return to work, fatigue, and qualitative and quantitative problems with their milk as troubles they experience with breast-feeding. Overweight nursing women experience these difficulties and then some. These range from trouble initiating a good milk flow to having technical difficulties with the infant's suckling at the breast. There are also some questions as to the quality of the milk. Some research suggests that the breast milk of obese women contains higher amounts of fat and lower amounts of protein, so any dietary protein deficit could possibly put some overweight moms' babies at risk for protein difficiency. However, this is currently a theoretical problem, not a clinical one, because, at least in this country, the protein content of a new mom's diet is usually high anyway.

In a study from Australia, obese women were found to be less apt to initiate breast-feeding. Furthermore, those who did breast-feed stopped sooner than their thinner counterparts. There are certain characteristics of women who tend to breast-feed longer, as we've heard before. These include:

• **Age:** Older mothers are more inclined to breast-feed longer than younger mothers.

• **Education:** The higher your level of education, the longer you tend to continue breast-feeding.

• **Economic Class:** The wealthier you are, the more likely you are to continue breast-feeding.

• **Relationships:** The more stable the relationship with the baby's father, the longer breast-feeding continues.

Finally, obese women are often afflicted with gestational diabetes and high blood pressure. Nursing moms with these two conditions are more inclined not to initiate nursing.

Nursing is a unique milestone in a woman's life. Just think about all your body and you have done over these past nine months or so just to be in a position to nurse! Yet I can't stress enough that your decision to breast-feed, and for how long, should never be based on guilt, or on fear of harming your baby if you don't. If it is something that you feel totally comfortable with, then do it; if not, don't. The message here is that any woman, no matter what she weighs, can always give nursing her best shot. Should you start nursing and find that it's just not the right fit for you, you can stop and switch to formula.

No one said that nursing is easy. To be good at something requires effort and the right attitude. Some of the technical difficulties cited above may come into play, but I am sure that you can overcome them if nursing means a lot to you. My advice? Try it—you might like it!

A WORD ABOUT SUPPLEMENTS

You know that nursing moms need more of everything: from increased protein to minerals such as calcium and magnesium. Review the chart on page 85, and you will notice that the Recommended Dietary Allowance for most vitamins and minerals is increased for nursing moms. For instance, calcium is especially important because the baby's growing skeleton needs lots of calcium, and it's either going to come from your food or from your skeleton! However, in order to obtain the minimum amount of vitamins and minerals that you now need from your food alone, you would have to consume at least 3000 calories a day. Overweight and obese moms should know that you don't lose weight eating 3000 calories per day: You gain weight! Therefore, the healthiest way to provide for your needs and still lose weight is by continuing a habit that you began before you conceived: take supplements. Be sure that the supplement that you are taking contains at the very least all of the necessary vitamins and nutrients shown on the chart on page 85. I recommend taking the more potent prescription pre-natal vitamins. Popping one pill full of what will make your baby grow and maintain your good health gives you one less thing to worry about!

If you aren't sure which supplement is best for you, ask a health professional. Pharmacists are an excellent resource for information on supplements. Keep in mind that more is not always better. The vitamins and minerals that you ingest find their way to your baby through your milk; and certain vitamins, such as vitamin A and vitamin D, as well as minerals such as selenium, may be harmful to your baby if you take doses higher than recommended.

Finally, supplements do just that: they supplement your food, not replace it!

MIXING WATER AND OIL

To fine-tune your weight loss experience while nursing, add two things to the mix: water and oil.

Water

If you are nursing, you need to drink more water than usual. Because the water you drink does not necessarily become part of the milk that you make, the old wives' tale that the more water you drink, the more milk you make has no basis in fact.

However, it is true that if you nurse, your body requires extra water while it produces milk. It is suggested that you increase your fluid intake up to two quarts a day, but I believe that your thirst mechanism should really dictate how much water you drink. If you force yourself to drink too much water, you can actually interfere with prolactin and reduce your milk production! Keep in mind that some foods, such as soups and vegetables, consist mostly of water, but fluids like juices and sodas, while also consisting mostly of water, add calories that you don't need. The safety of consuming diet drinks while breast-feeding is not known, and I don't recommend drinking large amounts of them. Water is ideal for breast-feeding moms. If you are the type of woman who doesn't like to drink a great deal of water, you should know that the foods you eat all contain varying amounts of water. The highest amounts are found in fruits such as watermelon; even a piece of cooked steak can contain up to 60 percent water. Always try to keep a big bottle of cool, refreshing water nearby. One mom we know sips on a large glass of water each time she nurses: when baby drinks, mom drinks, too!

Fish Oil

Almost every week, it seems, there is another news story extolling the virtues of fish oil for the prevention of heart attacks. After all, the Inuit, who eat whale and seal blubber that contains lots of fish oils, suffer fewer heart attacks than we do. What you may not know is that the Inuit have a higher incidence of plaque in their cerebral blood vessels and a higher incidence of strokes! But that's a story for a different day!

Anyway, the suggestion is out there for nursing women to increase the amount of a fish oil called *docosahexanenoic acid*, or DHA, in their diets. DHA is also known as an omega-3 fatty acid. It is believed by some (but not all) that this essential fatty acid, found in cold-water fish such as sole, mackerel, or cod, helps a baby's brain and eye development. Because of this, many nursing women and even some pregnant women take fish oil capsules as supplements. While it may turn out that this and other oils are beneficial, right now the data are scanty at best. Therefore, I believe that taking the fish oil capsules currently sold in health food stores may not be safe. These fish oil capsules enter your breast milk, and they contain high levels of the fat-soluble vitamins A and D. As we've noted, ingesting excessive amounts of these vitamins may affect your baby's health adversely. Also, you may already be getting the maximum dose of these vitamins from your daily food intake and supplements. A safer way to ingest omega-3 fatty acids is the natural way: by eating deep-sea fish, which are also a great source of the extra protein that you need.

Vegetable Oil

Recent research has shown that there is one type of oil that may help your baby's physical, and perhaps even mental, development during the first year of life. It is called *linoleic acid*, and it is known as an essential fatty acid. Linoleic acid is found in breast milk, and its content in breast milk is dependent on the amount of linoleic acid in mom's diet. Some new moms are deficient in this fatty acid. Good sources of linoleic acid are sunflower, peanut, sesame, and canola oils. Since you only need one tablespoon of linoleic acid per day, you can incorporate these oils in your cooking, or use them as salad dressings. It is interesting to note that commercial salad dressings that contain the oils mentioned above usually contain large amounts of linoleic acid. For example, Newman's Own Balsamic Vinaigrette is a good source of linoleic acid. Just be careful how much salad dressing you use! Some dressings are almost pure fat and contain lots of artery-clogging saturated fat and calories! One tablespoon should be enough!

A WORD ABOUT HERBS AND ALTERNATIVE REMEDIES

Nursing moms should not be ingesting herbal remedies. Herbs, including tea leaves, find their way into your milk, and their effects on your infant are not known. Until more research is done in this area, play it safe, and wait until you stop nursing before you resume taking alternative medications.

THE THIRD TRIMESTER OF WEIGHT LOSS: AN OVERVIEW

How much weight can an overweight or obese new mom who nurses expect to lose in the third weight loss trimester? If you notice, the eating plan for the third weight loss trimester differs little from the other two weight loss trimesters, qualitatively. The big difference is that the biochemical circumstances of the third weight loss trimester are perfect for overweight and obese new moms. They can eat more, exercise, and lose lots of weight! Keep in mind that if you are a Type B (overweight) or a Type C (obese) new mom, you tend to lose the most weight of all new moms, and breast-feeding amplifies your body's weight loss abilities. Your chances of weighing less than before you were pregnant are excellent! A review of the medical literature suggests that nursing moms should limit their weight loss to one pound per week, at least for the first few weeks. Would one pound per week satisfy you? This doesn't seem like a great deal of weight, but let's do some math. Should you nurse for six months, this translates to about 25 pounds of fat lost! If you nurse for nine months, your tally rises to about 35 pounds! However, we know from experience that many woman have lost twice these amounts.

The recommendation of losing one pound per week was based on the fear that thinner new moms, especially those in their teens, might try to lose too much weight and put the health of their nursing infants in jeopardy. Weight loss is an individualized process, and how much weight you lose will be determined by your own body chemistry and by how closely you follow the program in this book. However, if you are overweight or obese, I don't think that there should be any restrictions regarding your rate of weight loss, so long as you are providing adequate nutrition to your baby and yourself. To ensure this, I recommend that all overweight and obese new moms who nurse and who are

actively trying to lose weight should weigh in at their health professional's office every two weeks. You should let your obstetrician and
your child's pediatrician know that you are nursing and losing weight.
Both of these doctors will want to make sure that your baby is *gaining*
weight while you are *losing* weight!

ONE FINAL WEIGHT LOSS GIFT

For those of you who nurse, once you stop, nature presents you with a
final weight loss gift. As your body's milk-making apparatus shuts
down, your breasts shrink back to their normal size. You may not have
realized it, but all the time that you were nursing, the extra weight of
your breasts added about 5 pounds to your body weight. Now it's time
to get on the scale. You will be 5 POUNDS LIGHTER!

Part III

The Pregnancy
XL Files

Chapter Nine

Prepping for Your Next Pregnancy

Think of this section as a sneak preview, an advance screening, of your favorite movie. Some of you may plan to get pregnant again and others may be reading this book early in your pregnancy. You should know that there are two important factors of postpartum weight loss success that come to bear during your pregnancy: limiting the weight gain of pregnancy and coming to grips with the diabetes of pregnancy, or gestational diabetes. At first glance these factors may seem unrelated, but they are closely intertwined. Excess weight gain begets diabetes, and both can wreak havoc with postpartum weight loss. This does not mean that if you have gained a lot of weight and have gestational diabetes, you won't succeed at postpartum weight loss. *Hello, Baby! Good-bye, Baby Fat!* is based on the premise that the postpartum is the best time for *any* new mom to lose weight. Excess weight gain and gestational diabetes just make things harder for you, especially if you are a Type B (overweight new mom) or a Type C (obese new mom). Intuitively, you know that the more weight you carry, the harder it is to lose: Who has an easier chance of eventually weighing 135 pounds: a 225-pound new mom or a 150-pound new mom? The answer is obvious.

But what may not be apparent is that there is a lot you can do to prevent excessive weight gain during your pregnancy, minimize your risk of gestational diabetes, and make your postpartum weight loss that much easier. After all, *you* are in control!

THE MORE YOU GAIN, THE MORE YOU RETAIN

Pregnant women gain weight, right? Actually, some pregnant women gain *no* weight, and some women, especially if they are obese, *lose* weight during pregnancy—presumably because their bodies already contain enough adipose (fat) tissue to supply nourishment to the developing fetus without any further weight gain. For all of you other moms-to-be, just as sure as the sun comes up tomorrow and it *does* rain in Indianapolis in the summertime, you are going to gain weight. It's a fact of life.

As soon as that pink positive sign appears on your home pregnancy test, you ask yourself the same question that you will soon ask your doctor, "How much weight should I gain?"

Why all the fuss about weight? According to all the research that has been conducted over the past thirty years, the amount of weight that you gain during pregnancy is not only a big deal—it's a *huge* deal! In fact, the amount of weight you gain during pregnancy is a major factor in your postpartum success. The more weight you gain, the more weight you will retain afterward. The less weight you gain, the less you retain. If you need a slogan, you now have one: THE MORE YOU GAIN, THE MORE YOU RETAIN.

The scientific documentation for your new slogan is easy to find. Just take a quick look at the results of a large study published in the prestigious medical journal *Obstetrics and Gynecology* in March 1992. Seven hundred and ninety-five women who had recently delivered were divided into three groups based on the amount of weight they gained during pregnancy. The first group of mothers gained less then 25 pounds, the second group gained between 25 and 35 pounds, and the third group gained more than 35 pounds. When the researchers checked these women *six months* after delivery, they found that the women in the first group (those who gained less than 25 pounds during their pregnancies) weighed 2.6 pounds less than before they were pregnant! Those women who gained between 25 and 35 pounds in pregnancy were 3.5 pounds heavier than before pregnancy, and the women who gained over 35 pounds were now 11 pounds heavier! These dramatic results clearly show how important just a few pounds are at this crucial time. Interestingly, weight loss for almost all women in the three different groups came to a stop at six months, just as we have predicted in our new mom weight loss paradigm. This six-month window for weight loss is real, make no mistake about it!

Other studies suggest that when a "desirable-weight" American woman gains over 30 pounds during pregnancy, she will retain about 4 pounds at one year postpartum. Four pounds may not seem like a lot, but let's compare our situation with what occurs in Japan and you will see just what 4 pounds can mean. Japanese women gain, on average, about 23 pounds while pregnant, 7 pounds less than their American counterparts. After delivery, fully 85 percent of these women have returned to their pre-pregnancy weights! New moms in Japan weigh 7 pounds less while pregnant and retain 4 pounds less postpartum than the American women do! This is exactly what the studies predicted: the more you gain, the more you retain.

But there is much more to this 4-pound issue than just cosmetics. Japanese women have a far lower incidence of obesity, diabetes, high blood pressure, heart disease, and breast cancer than American women do. Those few extra pounds are not only harder to take off, but as little as 4 or 5 pounds can make the difference between becoming a diabetic, having high blood pressure, or developing heart disease. Every pound counts! And controlling the amount of weight you gain while pregnant becomes crucial in the prevention scheme. You can actually sabotage your weight loss efforts as a new mom by gaining too much weight during pregnancy. In fact, for many of you, the amount of weight you gain *while* pregnant is more important in determining your long-term weight prognosis than how much you weighed prior to pregnancy!

THE WEIGHT GAIN TIGHTROPE

All pregnant women walk a weight gain tightrope. They must balance the health of their baby with concerns about their own health and weight. The bottom line reads like this: The optimum maternal weight gain to ensure postpartum weight loss success is about 20 pounds. The optimum maternal weight gain to ensure your baby's proper growth and avoid problems at delivery is closer to 25 pounds. That's a 5-pound gap. Certainly, you want your baby to be healthy and grow to his or her maximum potential while inside you, but on the other hand you don't want to be saddled with a permanent weight gain. So how much should you weigh to satisfy your baby's health needs and your own? Moreover, how much weight should women gain who are overweight or underweight before getting pregnant?

After all, children born to either underweight and overweight mothers are at risk of having severe complications at delivery as well as future health problems.

This sounds like a conundrum worthy of King Solomon himself. With so much at stake, the American College of Obstetrics and Gynecology has been grappling with the issue of weight gain in pregnancy for decades. Recommendations regarding the optimum weight for a mom-to-be have gone up and down like a yo-yo.

In the 1920s, heaviness in children was equated with being robust and healthy. The heavier a woman and the more weight she gained during pregnancy, the larger (and presumably healthier) the baby. As a result, unlimited weight gain during pregnancy was the norm. By the 1930s, it was discovered that heavier women had more difficult labors and deliveries. They also had postpartum complications such as bleeding and diseases of the gallbladder and kidneys. Recommendations against unlimited weight gain were therefore implemented, but exact numbers were never furnished.

LESSONS LEARNED FROM HISTORY

Then came World War II, and with it we learned some incredible new information regarding the relationship between a mother's body weight and her child's health. Regrettably, though, this information was gathered at a terribly high price: the loss of human life.

Between September 8, 1941, and January 27, 1944, the German army blockaded the Russian city of Leningrad (now known as St. Petersburg). For 872 days, no food reached the city. Out of a population of 2.4 million, 1 million people died of starvation. The daily ration at this time was 300 calories per day, which is equivalent to the amount of calories in one chocolate bar! The diet Soviet moms ate consisted of vegetables, potatoes, and virtually no protein. Unbelievably, many women were still able to conceive. There was a high infant mortality rate, though, and the babies who survived were almost 20 percent smaller than normal babies. Later, I will tell you what happened to some of these babies.

This terrible experience repeated itself in Nazi-occupied Holland between October 1944 and May 1945, in what is known as the "Dutch famine." This time, pregnant women had to survive on less than 800 calories a day, due to food rationing. There was a high rate of still-births, and those babies who did survive were smaller than normal. Babies who were denied food during the third trimester suffered the most complications.

There were also thousands of recorded live births in concentration camps, prisons, and ghettos, where food was scarce. *Remember these suffering pregnant women and their babies of years past.* Today, as you will see, they give us valuable lessons for your health and that of your baby.

Based on the war experience, scientists realized that mothers did not have to gain lots of weight to ensure that their babies would be healthy, and weight gain recommendations were lowered. In the 1950s and 1960s, pregnant women were advised to gain between 15 and 20 pounds. With larger gains, it was thought, women ran the risk of a fluid buildup problem called preeclampsia and eclampsia, in which the mother develops dangerously high blood pressure. It was also believed that heavier moms delivered premature infants who had heart and lung complications. Doctors went far to enforce this weight limit, even requiring women over their weight limit to diet—*a major medical no-no!* Pregnant women should never, ever diet! Some were even prescribed powerful appetite suppressants, known as amphetamines, in order for them to lose weight. Again, this is a *major medical no-no!* Imagine, just a few short years ago, perhaps your mother, grandmother, or aunt was treated this way!

Now, fast-forward to the 1990s. We live in an industrialized world and eat a high-fat, low-nutrient diet, growing heavier and heavier each year. Obesity is epidemic, and it seems that a new sense of permissiveness regarding weight gain for moms-to-be has reappeared. The amount of pregnancy weight gain advocated by the medical community has been creeping up. I see plenty of obese women in my office who gained 40, 50, even 70 pounds with their pregnancies. Are we really back to the "Roaring Twenties" again, with almost *unlimited* weight gain the norm for pregnant women?

"I AM PREGNANT. HOW MUCH SHOULD I WEIGH?" THE ANSWER FOR THE MILLENNIUM

What is the perfect weight for a pregnant woman, to increase the odds of a healthy delivery and lifelong wellness for both her baby and her?

You already know that the answer to this question has changed many times in this century alone and will probably change again as research continues. In an effort to answer this important question, a task force of government and private-sector scientists studied the issue over several years. Based on their findings, new weight gain guidelines were issued in the early 1990s. These guidelines have become standard medical practice. Although many doctors do not follow them to the letter, these are the guidelines that your doctor uses to determine ideal maternal weight gain. They are medical science's attempt to answer a question that in reality has no one answer. There is no single perfect weight for pregnant women. A one-size-fits-all approach is out.

Each of you is unique. Whether you are a Type A, Type B, or Type C, you each have your own special set of weight gain characteristics. So instead of assigning one ideal weight for each new mom, scientists have developed a customized set of ideal weight *ranges* that are based on a woman's height and weight prior to pregnancy. It is hoped that these recommended weights provide the maximum health benefit for each new mom and her new baby. The underlying principle to the weight range guidelines is a simple one: IF YOU ARE PREGNANT, YOU SHOULD GAIN NEITHER TOO MUCH WEIGHT NOR TOO LITTLE.

Always keep in mind that these weights are to be used as guidelines, but they are not guarantees. Nature provides no guarantees!

Let's take a closer look at the guidelines. They are based on your height and weight. A number of years ago it was discovered that your height and weight are intertwined and can be factored together to give you an indication of how much fat you have on your body. This relationship is called the *body mass index*, or BMI. The body mass index can also be used as a predictor of your future health, whether you are pregnant or not. That's why the body mass index has replaced the old life insurance tables as the industry standard. The higher your BMI, the more body fat you have, and the more likely you are to experience weight-related illnesses, such as high blood pressure, diabetes, and some cancers. The BMI has even been used to predict longevity—the higher the BMI, the shorter the life span!

The BMI is used for pregnant women because of the important lessons we have learned from pregnant women throughout history. Your body type and pre-pregnancy weight, coupled with the amount of weight you gain during pregnancy, have a corresponding effect on your baby's birth weight. If your BMI is high, chances are high that you will give birth to a large baby. If your BMI is below the normal range, you may give birth to a below-normal-weight baby.

Ideally, then, by keeping the amount of weight gained during your pregnancy within recommended ranges, you can avoid the problems presented by the two extremes of being overweight or underweight. (Again, nature does not always cooperate, and keeping your weight within the recommended BMI range is not a guarantee against all the things that can go awry during the birthing process and postpartum.)

Amid all this technical talk, don't lose sight of what you are trying to do: lose weight after pregnancy. Your BMI is an important indicator in this regard. If your BMI is high before pregnancy, you should do all you can to limit your pregnancy weight gain. Doing so will make your postpartum weight loss that much easier. Even though the new pregnancy weight gain guidelines weren't developed with your postpartum weight loss in mind, you already know that THE MORE YOU GAIN, THE MORE YOU RETAIN.

Let's get going by figuring out your body mass index. Once you know your BMI, I will show you how much weight you should gain in pregnancy. A complex formula is used to determine your BMI, and you most certainly need a calculator, if not an advanced degree in math, to use it. To make things a bit easier, here is a "quickie" chart that lets you find your own BMI in a snap.

Locate your height in the far left column of the BMI chart. Look along the line of weight boxes to the right of your height and find the weight box that is closest to your pre-pregnancy weight. Then look down to the very bottom of the column that your weight box is in. That number is your BMI! The average American women stands 5'4" and weighs 145 pounds. If you check her BMI you will find it to be 25. Remember that your body mass index (BMI) is based on your weight prior to pregnancy.

Once you know your BMI, your next step is to find out how much weight you should gain during your pregnancy. It's as easy as looking at the following table, issued in 1992 by a 21-member commission of nutritionists, pediatricians, epidemiologists, and obstetricians at the Institute of Medicine. This table is used by your doctor when he or she recommends the amount of weight you should gain.

The Body Mass Index (BMI)

WEIGHT (pounds)

	BMI 19	20	21	22	23	24	25	26	27	28	29	30
H 4'11"	94	99	104	109	114	119	124	128	133	138	143	148
E 5'	97	102	107	112	117	122	128	133	138	143	148	153
I 5'1"	100	106	111	116	121	127	132	137	143	148	153	158
G 5'2"	103	108	114	119	124	130	136	142	147	153	158	164
H 5'3"	107	113	118	124	130	135	141	146	152	158	163	169
T 5'4"	110	115	121	127	133	138	145	151	157	163	169	174
5'5"	114	120	126	132	138	144	150	156	162	168	174	180
5'6"	118	124	130	136	143	149	155	161	167	173	179	185
5'7"	121	127	134	140	146	153	159	166	172	178	185	191
5'8"	124	130	137	143	150	156	164	171	177	184	190	197
5'9"	128	135	141	148	155	162	169	176	182	189	196	203
5'10"	133	139	146	153	160	167	174	181	188	195	202	209
5'11"	135	143	150	157	164	171	179	186	193	200	207	215
BMI	19	20	21	22	23	24	25	26	27	28	29	30

RECOMMENDED WEIGHT GAIN FOR PREGNANT WOMEN

1. **Underweight Women,** BMI of less than 19.8: 28–40 pounds
2. **Desirable-weight Women (Type A),** BMI 19.8–26: 25–35 pounds
3. **Overweight Women (Type B),** BMI 26–29: 15–25 pounds
4. **Obese Women (Type C),** BMI 29+: 15+ pounds

How did you do? If you are (or have been) pregnant, did you remain within these guidelines?

Most of the weight gained during your pregnancy is gained over the last two trimesters. This chart implies that a desirable-weight woman should gain about 1 pound a week during the last two trimesters; an underweight woman should gain about 1.25 pounds a week; and an overweight woman should gain about 0.7 pound per week. Obese women should gain about half a pound per week.

By the way, the definition of obesity in pregnancy is not as clear to the medical community as it should be. Some doctors define it as a pre-pregnancy weight of over 200 pounds, while others define it as a pregnancy weight of 200 pounds. The term "massive obesity" is reserved for those pregnant women weighing above 250 pounds. I think that it's a lot easier to determine obesity based on the above BMI chart. If your pre-pregnancy BMI is over 29, you are considered obese.

It is recommended that African-American women and teenagers strive for the upper end of a given range because studies show that African-American babies and babies born to teens are too often at the lower end of the birth weight curve. It is also felt that shorter women (under 5'2") should gain weight at the lower end of a given range, as these women are prone to having relatively large babies, which can lead to more complications at birth.

OBESE OR NOT OBESE?

Notice two other things about the pregnancy weight gain guidelines. First, underweight women should gain the most weight, and even they should limit their weight to 40 pounds! Second, while a 15-pound base weight gain is given for obese women, no upper limit is specified. There are insufficient data to make the proper weight gain determination at this point. The idea is to have obese women limit their weight gain to 15 pounds, which is still far under the recommended amount for normal-weight women. Some scientists feel that the upper limit for obese moms' weight gain should be 25 pounds. The reason for such stringent weight recommendations is that infants born to obese women who gain lots of weight have greater chances of life-threatening complications at birth.

Unfortunately, there are three weight-related issues that are not reflected well in the weight gain guidelines. The first is the problem with underweight teenage women, who often gain too little weight with their pregnancies. The second issue pertains to women who smoke; the third pertains to multiple births.

High School Moms

In this country, one out of every five teenage girls has had sexual intercourse by the time she is a junior in high school. Consequently, more than half a million babies are born each year to teenage mothers. We all know about the often horrific eating habits of teenagers—we were teenagers once ourselves! They feel they must be thin, often resulting in a distorted body image that can lead to eating disorders like bulimia and anorexia. After all, many of us were "there" once, too. Combine all of these factors and you have an increasing number of thin, unmarried teenage moms-to-be who don't eat nutritious food. It is not surprising that babies born to teenage mothers may suffer more birth-related complications and have lower birth weights.

Trying to educate pregnant teenagers to eat properly and make the necessary lifestyle changes to ensure healthy babies can be tough. Many girls in this situation try to hide their pregnancies for as long as possible by not gaining too much weight. Often, they avoid medical follow-up and, tragically, many of these girls do not even realize they are pregnant until the end of their pregnancies. I therefore make this appeal to you: If you or someone you know is pregnant and underweight (with a BMI under 20) or is a pregnant teenager, seek the care of a health professional with experience in this area. It may be a social worker, doctor, nutritionist, or psychologist, but please get help. These young women obsess about losing weight at a time when they should be gaining weight. This is not the time to worry about gaining weight and losing weight at the same time. It can't be done! Please get help.

Up in Smoke, Down on Smoke

Many teenagers and adults smoke, and I guess this is a good time to bring up the topic of smoking and pregnancy. I had hoped to avoid this topic because, honestly, it turns my stomach to talk about it. I am not being judgmental, but I recall recently seeing a late-term mom puffing away at the bus stop. I immediately conjured up a mental picture of the infant inside her taking a drag on a cigarette each time she does. It is an image a medical school professor impressed on me years ago, and I have never forgotten it. All of the harmful chemicals and toxins in cigarettes such as nicotine, carbon monoxide, tar, and carcinogens cross the placenta and go from the mother's blood right into the baby's! As if that weren't enough, remember that cigarettes contain cyanide. What kind of mother would give cyanide to a tiny baby? Not to mention the fact that women who smoke often give birth to smaller and sicker babies who have a 40 times greater risk of death at delivery or shortly after than babies born to nonsmoking mothers. New research has shown that even secondhand smoke can be harmful to a developing fetus.

I know that one out of every three women of childbearing age smokes. I also know how hard quitting can be. If you smoke and are trying to conceive, there are new strategies and medications that can help you kick the habit before you get pregnant. If you are pregnant and smoke, you also have options that should be discussed with your doctor. Weight gain upon smoking cessation is frequently a concern for those who are considering quitting. Those women who quit smoking just before becoming pregnant may gain an extra pound or two during their pregnancy, but they lose it just as quickly after delivery. There can be no disputing this one: Smoking during pregnancy is not worth it. You and your baby are worth more. Get help and quit now!

Twins, Triplets, and Beyond!

Notice that there are no pregnancy weight gain guidelines for twins, triplets, or other multiple births. That's because there are not many data available on which to base recommendations. About 2 percent of all births in the United States are twins. That's about 80,000 a year! There are approximately twelve hundred sets of triplets and eighty sets of quadruplets born each year, as well. Under ten sets of quintuplets and sextuplets are born and, as you well know from recent headlines, there has been one set of septuplets and one of octuplets.

This increase in multiple births is due to fertility drugs, in vitro fertilization and other cutting-edge techniques, and better overall medical care. Interestingly, a higher percentage of overweight and obese women give birth to twins than thinner moms.

Weight gain concerns for multiple birth moms are similar to those for underweight moms because low birth weight babies are the usual problem. Half of these babies are delivered prematurely and are at risk for developmental problems, such as lung and heart diseases. A current recommendation for moms pregnant with twins is a total weight gain of between 35 and 45 pounds. This translates to a weight gain of 1.5 pounds a week for the last two trimesters. If you are carrying multiple babies, make sure that you formulate an individual weight gain program with your doctor.

One study of twins suggests that to help ensure that each baby weighs over 5 pounds by the 37th week, you should gain 44 pounds during your pregnancy. Keep in mind that you and your babies require far more than single pregnancies do in terms of nutrition, especially if you decide to breast-feed. This, too, should be discussed with your doctor. Finally, the postpartum weight loss plan outlined in the book is valid for breast-feeding mothers of multiples, too, so long as nutrition is augmented accordingly. This can be done under the supervision of a nutritionist or another health care professional experienced in multiple births.

EATING FOR TWO: WHAT'S IN IT FOR YOU?

Now you know your BMI. Now you know how much weight your doctor will recommend that you gain with pregnancy. But what's really in it for you?

First of all, if you have exceeded your recommended weight gain, there is no need to worry or feel guilty. Anyone can lose weight after delivery. Pregnancy should be a time of joy, and worrying about excessive weight only detracts from this experience. Each of you has her own individual reasons for the how's and why's of weight gain during pregnancy. Of course, as you saw in Chapter Three, the weight you gain during pregnancy is driven biologically by the placental hormones of the baby, but that is not the end of the story. Personal and environmental factors, including eating habits, social pressures, the amount of food available, and attitude toward weight gain play major roles as well. No pregnant woman has complete conscious control over her weight gain, and she may feel pressure to eat (or not eat) from her family, her friends, and even her own doctor.

The messages are often conflicting and very confusing. The very same people who tell you not to gain too much weight may also be the first to offer you extra french fries and that last slice of pizza! Your doctor or nurse may remind you to eat enough for two, yet later may admonish you for gaining too much weight. The amount of pressure put on you at this vulnerable time is tremendous, but pregnancy is not the time to test your dieting resolve.

Under no circumstances should you ever try to lose weight while you are pregnant. It is possible that the breakdown products of fat cells, known as *ketones*, can interfere with your baby's development or even harm it. Dieting while pregnant must be considered unsafe because we are not sure of the implications for the baby.

EXTRA LARGE, EXTRA PROBLEMS

We know that weighing too little is not good, but what about weighing too much? From a purely obstetrical standpoint, excessive weight gain during pregnancy poses health risks for both you and your child during pregnancy, delivery, and the postpartum period. This discussion is not intended to scare you, but it cannot be ignored that there are certain problems that seem to plague the overweight and obese mom more than thinner moms, and I want you to know about them. Here they are.

HEALTH RISKS TO BABY

• **Macrosomia, or large body:** The more a mother weighs at delivery, the larger her baby will be. If the baby weighs over 8.8 pounds, it is considered to have macrosomia. Large babies can suffer from birth trauma and shoulder nerve damage (*dystocia*) as they pass through the birth canal. This nerve compression can lead to permanent paralysis. Large babies often require a cesarean or forceps delivery, which, of course, further increases the risks for complications to both mother and child.

• **Neural tube defect:** Children born to obese mothers are at risk for *spina bifida*, a malformation (or neural tube defect) involving the spinal column and spinal cord. This condition can cause severe permanent paralysis and even death. Until a few years ago, it was believed that neural tube defect was caused primarily by folate deficiency. Folate, or folic acid, is one of the B vitamins and is often deficient in our diets; this is why it is recommended that any women of childbearing age take a folic acid supplement. Unfortunately, it is now known that obesity by itself poses a risk factor for this serious neurological disorder.

• **Future health risks:** Large babies are more apt to develop diabetes and high blood pressure, and to become obese themselves.

HEALTH RISKS TO MOTHER

• **Hypertension:** Obese pregnant women are at higher risk for high blood pressure during pregnancy *and* afterward.

• **Diabetes:** The risk of gestational diabetes (the diabetes of pregnancy) is greatly increased in obese women (see Chapter Ten). Obese moms are also prone to diabetes later in life.

• **Increased incidence of kidney disease.**

• **Increased incidence of phlebitis,** a painful inflammation of the veins in the legs.

• **Increased incidence of gallbladder disease.**

• **Increased incidence of wound infection after a cesarean section:** Studies have shown that up to 15 percent of all cesareans done on obese women have become infected, some seriously.

• **Obese moms have more bleeding complications** and an increased chance of blood clots should they need surgery after delivery.

• **Obese women have prolonged labor and more difficult deliveries in general.**

This list would not be complete without the final health risk: excessive maternal weight gain. The more weight you gain with your pregnancy, the more weight you will retain after delivery, and the higher your risk for obesity later in life. This holds true whether or not you were thin prior to pregnancy. However, there is hope: Controlling the amount of weight gain with this pregnancy, no matter how much weight you gained with a previous pregnancy, can dramatically enhance your future weight loss success. So many women do not realize this and become resigned to being overweight after delivery when they don't have to—if they only implement the simple weight loss guidelines that you know about now!

PREGNANCY: THE NINE-MONTH FEAST

My approach to gaining weight during pregnancy is simple. Staying within the suggested weight ranges must never be a chore or something that detracts from the wonderful experience of pregnancy. You have enough to think about at this time. Anyway, the whole issue of weight loss can be such a downer—who really wants to talk or think about that? But wait, there's a distinction to be made here. The discussion is not about weight loss; it is about limiting the amount of weight gain, and that makes all the difference in the world.

Was there ever a time in your life when you could feel so good about gaining weight? I doubt it. This, then, is a unique *weight gain* opportunity for you, so take advantage of it. Imagine, for a moment, that you are invited to a large tropical feast. You can eat anything you want and as much as you want. With no limits imposed you really go to town, eating everything in sight. The next morning you wake up with that, "I'll never eat another morsel of food" feeling. You overdid it . . . all that food actually made you sick to your stomach. You vow never to eat that much again and to stay away from tropical feasts. A year passes and you are invited to the same feast again. Of course, you go. With last year's memories etched in your mind, this time you eat the same foods, but in smaller portions. This time you feel great the next morning and you look forward to next year's feast. You've had a totally positive experience.

Pregnancy is a nine-month feast: You can eat the foods you enjoy and gain weight, yet you can feel good about yourself because you did it all in a healthy fashion. Never use your pregnancy as an excuse to eat everything on the table. You are not "eating for two"—I can't stand that expression. You should be eating healthily for two.

Having two doughnuts, two ice creams, or two pieces of cake does nothing for you *or* your baby; you both need nutritious foods. Studies are clear on this point: There are no known benefits to eating yourself past the recommended pregnancy weight gain guidelines. Common sense and a scale tell us that the idea that bigger is better is unhealthy. Quantity for quantity's sake is out. You need quality instead.

Remember those starving mothers in World War II? Those women didn't have enough to eat enough for *one*, yet they still bore a relatively high percentage of healthy, albeit smaller, babies. What became of some of these babies?

A fascinating follow-up study on babies born during that terrible siege of Leningrad was published in 1997 in the *British Medical Journal*. One hundred and sixty of those babies, now adults, were screened for diseases possibly associated with being born to starving mothers. It was theorized that since so much of a baby's in utero development depends on the nutritional status of the mother, starvation would cause structural problems to major organs, resulting in health problems in adulthood. Amazingly, no major medical problems were found, even though the subjects' mothers, under extreme stress, consumed only 300 calories per day and lacked proper medical attention. The majesty of a mother-child bond was never more clear. Somehow, a mother's body can shield her unborn child from the ravages of starvation. This may be a radical example of malnutrition, but it proves that overnutrition is not proper nutrition.

We are surrounded by food. In a sense we are under a siege of too much food! I still have confidence that you can do it. You know that unless you are underweight, there are no advantages in gaining a great deal of weight during pregnancy. You also know that excess weight gain can compromise your health and that of your baby, while making your postpartum weight loss efforts much more difficult. Intervening now, during pregnancy, is the healthy choice.

A pilot study was conducted at the University of Pittsburgh to see if properly supervised pregnant women could limit their weight gain to the recommended limits. Researchers established a three-pronged program of education, exercise, and low-fat diet. Three out of four normal-weight pregnant women in the program kept their weight at the recommended level. These women did it, and so can you! It does not require huge lifestyle changes. *Preventing* weight gain is much easier than losing weight, remember? Besides, pregnancy is not the time to start making sweeping changes in your diet. It is much easier—and more beneficial—to make small dietary adjustments now and reap the benefits later.

Let's go trimester by trimester to see which small adjustments can be made to your diet and lifestyle so that you can exert control over your pregnancy weight gain. Keep in mind that if you are underweight or if you have medical problems such as diabetes (see Chapter Ten), you should be under the care of a medical doctor and a nutritionist, and you should not follow these dietary suggestions without their approval.

FIRST TRIMESTER: LIMITING WEIGHT GAIN

Once your doctor knows that you are pregnant, he or she will give you two things: a prescription for prenatal vitamins and information sheets regarding which foods you should be eating. Make certain that you take your vitamins every day. You need extra vitamins and minerals such as folate and iron, and supplements are an easy way to make sure you get the necessary amounts. Keep in mind that more is not better here, either. Taking too much vitamin A, vitamin D, or selenium may harm your baby, so just take what the doctor ordered!

More than likely you will pick up a book about nutrition and pregnancy. It seems like the thing to do, especially for first-time moms, and there are many good ones out there. Books and information sheets have their place, but they all have one big flaw—they are not personalized for the "real" you. Keep in mind that for centuries women of all cultures have eaten pretty well by trusting their instincts, without the benefit of these resources, and so can you. It is interesting to note that veteran moms rarely buy these books because, after the first or second child, they realize something that I am sharing with you right now. These books often presume that you are going to be a "food saint"—someone who makes only the healthiest choice each and every time she eats (e.g., substituting carrots for chocolate). A food saint never eats ice cream but chooses low-fat yogurt instead. She will eschew cakes and cookies for whole wheat crackers. Then there is the "real" you. The "real" you knows she should have yogurt but loves ice cream too much to give it up. The "real" you has the good intention of eating more fruits and veggies, but winds up giving in to Kit Kat bars more often than not. In Chapter Three, you learned that your cravings for high-fat foods are biologically driven, so your food choices are not entirely your own. Therefore, let's inject some realism into the scheme of things. You don't have to be a saint, making perfect, healthy food choices over the next nine months. You need to fashion a style of eating that is comfortable for the "real" you. All you need is faith in yourself, common sense, and a scale.

THE MORNING HEAVE-HO

Weight gain is usually minimal in the first trimester. Don't worry if you look down and there is no belly in sight. You may not gain any weight over the first few weeks. Some women actually lose weight in the early weeks because of the nausea and vomiting associated with morning sickness. About one half of all pregnant women experience morning sickness, which in fact can strike at any time of day and last for months. There are a few things you should know about morning sickness and the early part of the first trimester, in general. There is absolutely no reason to force-feed yourself. Eat when and if you are hungry. It does no harm to your developing baby if you do not gain weight now. In early pregnancy, the fetus is microscopic in size and takes several weeks to attain the size of a grain of rice. Your baby does not require a great deal of nutrition now. The needs of the fetus are more than met by the food that you consume, even if you have morning sickness.

For some women, certain foods can act as triggers for their nausea and vomiting spells, so take notice and stay away from them. Often, just the smell of these foods can set you off. Some doctors advocate eating high-protein and high-carbohydrate meals before your next onset of nausea to offset the symptoms, while others recommend taking an extra dose of vitamin B_6. Check with your own doctor. Above all, don't try any fad diet that purports to alleviate morning sickness; there is no such diet. Some women swear they solved their stomach problems by drinking spearmint tea mixed with half a teaspoon of ginger. Others found success by drinking chamomile tea. Who knows? Morning sickness will abate by itself; just be patient. It is almost a normal part of being pregnant. Don't try and outeat it!

Pregnancy affects your thirst mechanism too. You will eventually find yourself extremely thirsty and apt to drink the first beverage that you can find. Be prepared and beat your thirst to the punch by having lots of cold water readily available This way you will avoid the empty calories of soft drinks. I think that pregnant women should avoid drinking diet drinks, as their safety record in pregnancy is unknown.

PICKLES, ICE CREAM, AND MORE PICKLES

Having unusual cravings—the "pickles and ice cream syndrome"—is part of the first trimester, although it may persist even longer. Hormones play a definite role in cravings, which are usually for high-fat or salty foods (or both, as in the case of potato chips). Again, there is no reason to be a food saint. You can try to hold out for as long as possible, but you will probably give in to temptation sooner or later. You may as well have a plan to control these cravings before they hit. I believe in confronting, not avoiding, them.

First of all, never skip meals. When you skip a meal, your body chemistry demands that you eat more later, making you hungrier and more likely to crave food than before. Decide what foods are your favorite snacks and keep a small amount of them on hand. I consider them emergency junk foods. They should be the smallest serving size possible. Avoid buying large multi-packs or family-sized snack foods. Instead of feeling guilty because you crave foods, eat them! That's right, eat them! In my experience, women who nibble all day on small, fat-free snacks take in far more calories than do those who just give in to their needs but do it judiciously. The whole mind game that is played out over a little piece of chocolate cake or ice cream can be depressing and self-defeating. Empowering the food that you crave just makes its lure that much stronger. As time passes, you crave the food so much that you eat far more of it than you might if you simply give in and eat some when you first feel the craving. You also enjoy it much less than if you had eaten the food when the craving first hit.

I like to use the "rule of one." Your daily snack—and you can probably have two of these—should consist of one of anything: *one* chocolate bar, *one* scoop of ice cream, or *one* small bag of potato chips. You start to get into trouble when you reach for handfuls of food with no predetermined portions. Get used to eating a single unit of your favorite snack food. Eat *one*, enjoy *one*, and be content with *one*.

Some women notice that their sense of smell becomes more acute during pregnancy. Odors that you never even paid attention to before may now dominate your food choices. This heightened sensitivity to scents is hormonally induced. Be prepared when you go to the bakery or the supermarket—your enhanced sense of smell may wreak havoc on your appetite. Know what you are buying before you go in; have a list ready and stick with it. Don't be led around by your nose.

Get used to eating in one place only: the kitchen. Avoid eating in front of the television, in your bedroom, or in the living room. This habit will serve you well after you deliver, too. Just think how often your favorite T.V. shows are interrupted by commercials advertising food that looks perfect, while an announcer tells you just how perfect it tastes. By avoiding T.V. while eating, we avoid all those nasty subliminal and not so subliminal messages. When you do watch T.V. make sure you have eaten before you get comfortable.

Learn how to do the cabinet/refrigerator shuffle. Everyone has junk in their attics and basements, perhaps potential garage sale rejects. Make sure that the same can't be said about your kitchen. Outside of your little stash that we talked about, start throwing away all the stuff that can cause your downfall and may not even really taste that good. Get rid of all those bottles of condiments that you haven't used in years; they are the worst calorie offenders around! Many of you would be shocked if you read the labels on salad dressings to see how much fat they contain.

That can of whipped cream that hasn't been touched in the last seven months, and is probably rusty inside—out it goes. Where are your fresh fruits and vegetables? Start giving them front-row preference. Take them out of their lonely bins so that every time you open the fridge, they're right there in all their glory. Then at least you have a fighting chance to snack healthier. If you have children in the house, it will serve them well to eat better, too. Don't use other people in your household as an excuse to buy your favorite snacks. Make this a family thing; everybody should be eating healthier now!

Those of you who like to exercise should continue to do so, under medical supervision. Some of you who are not used to daily exercise may want to begin now. Multiple studies have shown that regular exercise during pregnancy can not only limit your weight gain but cause you to have easier labor, less incidence of back pain, fewer varicose veins, and less constipation. Your health care professional will be glad to furnish you with proper instructions and guidelines for your prenatal exercise program. Often local community centers, spas, and churches offer exercise programs for pregnant women. Just make sure that you obtain medical clearance from your doctor before undertaking any exercise program.

THE SECOND TRIMESTER

Your baby is getting big. By the start of the fourth month, a fetus is about four inches long and has fingers and toes. You are getting bigger too, and that's fine. We hope that the morning sickness has disappeared. The placenta is now producing hormones to make you hungry, and your appetite is increasing. That's fine, too, and perfectly normal, because it is estimated that the average pregnant woman needs an extra 300 calories per day.

At this point, you may start to "show" and the whole world finally knows that you are pregnant. Overweight or obese women with modest weight gains, especially those with a pear or hourglass shape, will show less. Those shaped like apples, carrying their weight in the abdominal area, will show more.

Be prepared: The first thing that many people are going to do is offer you food. People probably won't be offering you a roasted chicken and whole wheat crackers. More than likely they will be offering you the same types of things that they would offer you on Christmas, or birthdays—cakes, cookies, and potato chips. They think that you are eating for two and they represent society's wish to fatten you up. This is a "no-brainer." Learn to say "no." In times of doubt, just remember that if it is unhealthy for a full-sized adult to be overweight, could it be any less unhealthy to give a developing fetus all those empty calories? Just say no, because you care.

Learn to say "yes" to the recommendations that your doctor and nutritionist make. Most likely they will suggest meals that are largely based on complex carbohydrates and protein, including low-fat dairy products, keeping fat to a minimum. This middle-of-the-road approach works well for both baby and you. However, portion control is the key. Studies have shown that overweight women tend to underestimate their food intake by one half! For instance, when overweight women are asked to do a calorie count of daily intake, they may guess 1500 when it's really 3000! Some of the confusion lies in the definition of a serving size. What does one ounce of peanut butter look like, or an ounce of fish or potato salad? How about bagels, everyone's morning staple these days? One bagel can contain 300 calories, while another gigantic bagel contains 600! I personally use the "palm" rule. In general, one serving of any one solid food should fit in the palm of your hand. A bagel that is bigger than your palm is not one serving! Whenever you see a serving size listed on a package of food, look at your palm and decide if the amount listed is the amount you want or need.

Snack *smart*. Start developing your own snacking system by incorporating some healthy choices. It's still fine to follow the snacking recommendations from trimester one, but you should be combining these with fresh fruit, whole wheat products, and yogurt. The operative word for any and every snack is portion control. If you can't control the amount you eat of a particular snack, switch to one that you can control. I have created my own list of favorite snacks which are delicious, relatively low in fat, and filling. Try them!

MY THREE FAVORITE COOKIES

• *Reduced Fat Oreo Cookies:* about 40 calories and 1 gram of fat per cookie
• *Keebler Fudge Shoppe Reduced Fat Fudge Stripe Cookies:* about 40 calories and 1.5 grams of fat per cookie
• *Nabisco Fat Free Peach Apricot Newtons Cobblers:* 60 calories, no fat per cookie

MY THREE FAVORITE ICE CREAMS

• *Edy's No Sugar Added Black Cherry Vanilla Swirl Light Ice Cream:* ½ cup contains 90 calories, 3 grams of fat
• *SnackWell's Low Fat Ice Cream Sandwiches:* 90 calories, 1.5 grams of fat
• *Healthy Choice Cappuccino Chocolate Chunk Low Fat Ice Cream:* ½ cup, 120 calories, 2 grams of fat

MY THREE FAVORITE CAKES

• *Entenmann's Light Fudge Brownies:* 1 strip contains 130 calories, 2.5 grams of fat

• *Entenmann's Light Golden Loaf Cake:* 1 serving has 130 calories, 0 grams of fat
   • *Snackwell Streusel Squares:* 150 calories, 3 grams of fat

Remember, low-fat does not mean license to finish the whole box. Moderation rules.

Get a hobby. Many women eat out of boredom. Sitting around watching TV is far less fun than developing that hidden musical or artistic talent. Learn a new skill, a new language, or how to play the piano. Make this time special for you, the mom-to-be.

THE THIRD TRIMESTER

During the final twelve weeks, the homestretch (and I mean stretch), your baby triples in size. Interestingly, this is when your baby starts getting his or her own fat deposits! Your appetite already will have peaked, and it begins to slow in the few weeks before delivery. As your body gets bigger, you slow down. This is how your body conserves energy for the birth of your baby. Your metabolic rate starts to rise now, and it accounts for an extra 200 calories burned per day.

By this time, your pregnancy eating habits are probably already a part of you and, if you followed our suggestion to eat what you like in moderation, then there should be no food that you crave after delivery. Good for you! Unless you have not gained enough weight, there is no reason to play catch-up now. Studies show that if you are a desirable-weight pregnant woman, eating more now does nothing to help your baby grow—it only serves to make *you supersized!* This is your body's way of protecting your child. If everything that you ate contributed to the baby's growth, the baby would weigh 20 to 30 pounds, making delivery an impossibility. Nature has apportioned a finite amount of your food to your baby, and the rest gets deposited on your body!

By now you should be getting a bit tired doing your everyday activities as you and your body anticipate labor. I do hope that you followed the regimen of high complex carbohydrate/low fat eating that your health care professional suggested, because this regimen helps combat fatigue.

Something else very interesting is taking place in your body now.

The enzyme that pushes fat into fat cells, fat lipase, becomes very active in the third trimester. This makes it all too easy for you to deposit fat. In fact, this is probably the easiest time in a woman's life for fat to be deposited on her hips and thighs. Keep this in mind when you make your food choices in the third trimester. Low fat is the mantra now.

Because you are so fatigued, it becomes increasingly difficult to stand and prepare meals. In our society, fast food and takeout foods seem like the answer to a third trimester woman's prayers. And I don't blame you. Who wants to stand around preparing meals for the family when your legs feel as though you are wearing iron boots? Help is just a phone call away; any type of food can be delivered around the clock. For instance, a strip mall just opened near my house. It boasts five shops: a pizzeria, a doughnut shop, a deli, a Chinese restaurant, and (you'll love this one) a Weight Watchers! Go figure! Since fast food has become a staple that many pregnant women rely upon, beginning on page 235 you will find the menus of the most popular fast-food restaurants broken down into the total amount of calories and fat calories of each item. There are also "best of" and "worse of" lists based on fat calorie content, and some surprises await you there. I feel that an occasional foray to a fast-food restaurant is fine, but don't get ambushed by making choices that have the highest fat content.

Keep in mind what we said about your fat enzyme: It's just waiting to snap up any extra fat from your diet, like a crocodile lying beneath the murky river waters, and stow it in your fat cells. Low-fat eating is more important now than ever.

The sandman also contributes to weight gain in the third trimester. Sleep disturbances are common, as the increased size of your stomach can interfere with normal sleep patterns. Abnormal sleep patterns, as you know from our discussion of postpartum depression (page 61), can lead you to eat more. Worse still, they may cause you to eat late at night or into the early morning hours. Make certain that you never go to bed without having eaten dinner, and try not to nap too close to your regular sleep time. In fact, try to go to bed a bit earlier now. Don't be afraid to ask a spouse or family member to put other children to bed. You need sleep!

Be sure to keep a full glass of water at your bedside. It is common for women in this trimester to get up to use the bathroom or to be thirsty at night. Rather than going to the kitchen and encountering all those food temptations, keep a drink ready by your bed.

WHAT'S EATING YOU?

No matter what trimester you are in, you may be eating all the right foods, watching your portions, and still gaining too much weight. Let's do some troubleshooting and see if we can find your problem. First, make certain that each time you weigh yourself, you use the same scale, and that the scale is accurate. I have seen doctors' scales vary by up to 10 pounds! Also, try to wear the same type of clothing each time you weigh in, especially during the winter months. Second, some medical problems can cause you to gain weight above and beyond the norm during pregnancy. Here are seven questions that will help determine whether your excessive weight gain may be medically based. Your doctor should address each:

1. Do you have a medical condition, such as thyroid disease or diabetes?
2. Did you quit smoking recently?
3. Do your fingers and feet feel "tight"? You may have edema, or fluid buildup.
4. Might you be carrying twins or triplets?
5. Has your physical activity diminished due to fatigue, depression, or other problems?
6. Has your eating increased due to boredom, depression, or social pressure?
7. Do you have an eating disorder, like bulimia?

Any of these seven questions answered in the affirmative can mean a large weight gain for you. If you feel that any of these scenarios pertains to you, please see your doctor immediately. Most of these problems can be corrected in short order.

Finally, controlling your weight can be difficult at *any* time. During pregnancy, with hormones helping your appetite along, it is no easier. However, you are in a unique situation. You aren't supposed to lose weight, or even maintain your weight. Your goal is to gain weight! Try to do it in a healthy manner. I know you can.

No matter what you weigh today, you will still be a weight loss success after delivery. Take it to heart that you did the best you could and feel good about yourself. After all, a new baby is about to join you on your journey through life. What better achievement could you have hoped for?

Chapter Ten

The Sweet Life: Avoiding Gestational Diabetes

Your pregnancy should be the sweetest nine months of your life; however, for many new moms, things become a bit *too* sweet! Each year, 150,000 pregnant women without previous medical problems discover that they have a unique form of diabetes. It is known as *gestational diabetes*, or the diabetes of pregnancy. Diabetes is a metabolic disorder involving the body's inability to utilize the hormone insulin appropriately. This causes blood sugar to rise to dangerously high levels. Gestational diabetes differs from the two other forms of diabetes, juvenile and adult-onset. While pregnant women may be afflicted with one of the other forms of diabetes, gestational diabetes by definition applies to women who contract the disease only during pregnancy. However, because gestational diabetes affects two people at the same time (you and your baby) I call it "team diabetes."

Controlling and possibly preventing this sugary downer is your final success factor for postpartum weight loss, because overweight gestational diabetics with the highest blood sugars rarely lose weight after delivery. In fact, they often become obese and develop adult-onset diabetes within a few years of giving birth! Their children are not at an increased risk for developing juvenile diabetes, but what happens to them as adults is a different story. Within certain ethnic groups, such as Native Americans and Hispanics, the chances that a child born to an affected mother will later develop adult-onset diabetes are quite high. Many scientists believe that with further research, this disturbing trend will be found in all ethnicities.

All is not bleak, though. There is a great deal that you can do to protect yourself and your baby from contracting gestational diabetes, so that in many cases it can be prevented. The best way to prevent gestational diabetes is by sensible weight gain in pregnancy.

Gestational diabetes is not rare, affecting about 3 to 5 percent of all pregnant women each year. That's how we arrive at the figure of 150,000 new cases diagnosed each year in this country. Gestational diabetes is a serious worldwide health problem, with new cases numbering in the millions. India, Arab nations in the Mediterranean region, and most of Southeastern Asia have extremely high rates of gestational diabetes. In our own country, gestational diabetes is three times more common in the Hispanic and African-American populations. Within the black community, those of Caribbean descent have the highest incidence. The bottom line is that no woman is immune, but there are known risk factors that increase your chances of developing the disease. You need to become familiar with them. If you have any of these risk factors, there is an excellent chance that you will develop gestational diabetes—and possibly adult-onset diabetes later on. Adult-onset diabetics run the risk of blindness, kidney failure, severe heart disease, and strokes. This is very serious business. I emphasize the risks not to scare you, but rather as a call to action. This begins by understanding the changes that take place in your body that lead to this metabolic mayhem.

While the exact cause of gestational diabetes is unknown, there is a link to the growth of the baby inside you. Rather than blame the baby, though, you should thank the baby. He or she is trying to warn you about the future of your health and give you some time to do something about it. The fact of the matter is, if you are overweight and have some of the risk factors that follow, you are likely to develop adult-onset diabetes anyway. The pregnancy may just give you a forewarning years in advance! It is much easier and healthier to prevent adult-onset diabetes than it is to treat it. By the time you are diagnosed, chances are you will already have damage to the blood vessels of the eyes, heart, brain, and kidneys.

Just ask Karen M., a 34-year-old mother, who is sitting in my office holding her 2-year-old son Justin on her lap. Karen gained 55 pounds with her pregnancy and developed gestational diabetes. At delivery, Karen weighed 222 pounds, and she lost only 15 pounds in the following year. Later, she would gain another 5 pounds and hover at a weight of 210 pounds. Karen had her genetic history, a case of postpartum depression, and gestational diabetes pitted against her weight loss efforts. In addition, she did not exercise or do anything else to aid her weight loss until four months after her delivery, which was when her postpartum depression was diagnosed. Keeping in mind the six-month weight loss window that we discussed earlier, we can already see that Karen unknowingly sabotaged her own weight loss.

Karen told me that a routine blood test performed in her second trimester revealed the telltale high blood sugar of gestional diabetes. She had had no symptoms, which is common, and no complications during labor, and she had been told that her body would return to normal—without diabetes—after delivery. Her doctor said there was nothing to worry about! As I listened, shocked at her doctor's attitude, I did my best to practice restraint. My mind filled with all the possible risks, and I was ready to enlighten her about the true situation at hand and the warning sign her gestational diabetes had given her. Karen was unaware that she, like all women with gestational diabetes, has an ultra-high risk of developing adult-onset diabetes and all of its complications later in life.

You need to have a higher degree of readiness than Karen if you're going to meet the challenge of gestational diabetes head-on. It begins with discovering whether you have the following risk factors for gestational diabetes.

GESTATIONAL DIABETES: WHO'S AT RISK?

Any woman can contract gestational diabetes, but here are the key risk factors:

• **Gestational diabetes with a previous pregnancy:** you have a 2 out of 3 chance of recurrence.
• **Family history:** having a parent or sibling with gestational or adult-onset diabetes.
• **Age:** the risk increases at ages above 30. The older you are, the higher the risk.
• **Macrosomia (large body):** you, or a previous child, weighed over 8 pounds, 8 ounces at birth.
• **Glycosuria (sugar in the urine):** you had a urine test that showed sugar present in your urine.

- **Hypertension:** you had high blood pressure at any time in your life.
- **Problems with a previous birth:** anyone who has experienced certain complications with a previous birth, including stillbirth.
- **Ethnicity:** African-Americans, Hispanics, Arabs, and Southeastern Asians are at higher risk.

The number one risk factor, however, is *being overweight!* It's really quite simple: the more you weigh before your pregnancy, and the more weight you gain with your pregnancy, the higher your risk of gestational diabetes. You don't have to be obese to bring on gestational diabetes.

Excess fat on your body can interfere with the way that the insulin in your body controls the amount of sugar in the blood. The level of sugar has to be just right. Levels that are either too high or too low present health problems. When the extra fat on your body prevents insulin from doing its job of lowering blood sugar (this is known as *insulin resistance*), your blood sugar levels increase, eventually spilling over into your baby's blood. The baby's pancreas then has to work overtime to produce enough insulin to keep up with all of the sugar that's coming from you. Your body makes more insulin, too, sometimes three times the normal level. The increase in insulin is called *hyperinsulemia*. All of this extra insulin floating around can have profound effects on your baby's health at birth, such as:

- **Large babies:** While we all want to have large, healthy babies, babies born to moms with gestational diabetes often get too large, usually weighing more than 8 pounds, 8 ounces. This is referred to as macrosomia, or large body, and can lead to serious birth trauma for both mom and baby. Remember, bigger does not always mean healthier.
- **Low blood sugar, or hypoglycemia:** Excess insulin lowers the baby's blood sugar. This can be a medical emergency requiring intravenous glucose. The baby's central nervous system is extremely sensitive to not having enough blood sugar.
- **Severe respiratory problems at birth:** Affected babies often require oxygen and respiratory treatment.
- **Yellow discoloration of the eyes and skin,** called jaundice.
- **Low calcium levels, or hypocalcemia:** This can be dangerous to a newborn's heart and muscles.

• **Blood disorders:** The baby's blood has the potential to become too thick.

• **Higher than normal risk of infant death at delivery and immediately following if diabetes goes untreated:** This is obviously the most feared complication of gestational diabetes. A new and increased awareness of this disease has brought mortality rates of babies with diabetic mothers down to almost the same level as rates for normal babies, provided that a diagnosis is made and treatment is provided during pregnancy.

Newer research has uncovered two more complications that these children may suffer later in life:

• **Obesity:** These large babies are more apt to be overweight as children and as adults.

• **Adult-onset diabetes:** These babies are at risk for developing adult-onset diabetes, which has a 90 percent association with obesity. That is, 9 out of every 10 adult-onset diabetics are obese! It all starts in the womb.

Remember, even if your last pregnancy was totally normal, you are still at risk, *especially if you gained a lot of weight between pregnancies!* Be certain to give your doctor a thorough genetic history and review the risk factors, one by one, with your obstetrician.

With all these current and future health problems riding on the presence of diabetes, how will you know if you have it? There is no need for high-tech diagnostic tests. A basic blood test, the oral glucose tolerance test, suffices. It's simply a blood test drawn after you eat some sugar. If this test gives a positive result, then a confirmational full-glucose tolerance test is done. Your doctor compares your blood sugar with a standardized chart of abnormal blood sugars, and if your value matches the chart, it is presumed that you have gestational diabetes. Because a urine test for blood sugar is not considered accurate during pregnancy, it is not used. Most doctors automatically screen for gestational diabetes between weeks 24 and 28 of your pregnancy. In high-risk groups, such as women who had gestational diabetes in a previous pregnancy, your doctor may want to start the screening process at weeks 16 through 20. Unless definite symptoms are present, testing is not done sooner because gestational diabetes usually develops at the end of the second trimester.

Many women experience some of the symptoms of gestational diabetes but mistakenly attribute them to normal symptoms of pregnancy because most of the symptoms overlap. Just take a look at these:

- fatigue
- excessive thirst
- increased urination
- frequent nighttime urination
- urinary tract infections
- vaginal yeast infections

The only true way to tell the difference is through a blood test. Make sure that you are properly screened—it's your responsibility! Many people are under the misconception that a change in dietary cravings, such as an increased desire for sugar, is an indicator of gestational diabetes. This is not true; there are no studies to prove that gestational diabetics crave sugar any more or less than women who are not diabetics do.

If you are diagnosed with gestational diabetes, go to the library and learn as much as you can about it. Your doctor will probably give you dietary instructions and exercise recommendations, and, in severe cases, may give you a home glucose monitor so you can track your glucose levels. Most women do not require insulin treatment and, because of the potential for harm to the baby, diabetic pills are not used. Diet is the treatment of choice, based on recommendations of both the American Diabetes Association and the American College of Obstetricians and Gynecologists. Typically, diet recommendations are based on percentages of macronutrients, such as 50 percent complex carbohydrates, 25 to 30 percent protein, and 25 percent fat calories per day. These amounts, however, must be individualized to your body weight, your personal lifestyle, and the absence or presence of other diseases, and of course must follow any fluctuations in your blood sugar level. The diet you will receive is not intended for weight loss. The goal, instead, is to maintain the health of you and your child by keeping both of your blood sugars at normal levels to avoid the complications cited earlier. Because diet is a key treatment of gestational diabetes, I strongly recommend that any woman diagnosed with gestational diabetes see a nutritionist for treatment. Again, you need individualized and specific care recommendations. This is no time for a "one-size-fits-all" approach. Remember, DO NOT TRY TO LOSE WEIGHT IF YOU DISCOVER YOU HAVE GESTATIONAL DIABETES. The breakdown products of fat cells, ketones, may interfere with your baby's development and could be very harmful to your child. You will have plenty of time to lose weight after delivery!

So, if you have gestational diabetes, or are at risk for developing it, what can you do to help yourself? Plenty! Your ally, and diabetes' Public Enemy Number One, is weight control. Studies show that as little as a 5- to10-pound weight loss can make the difference between a person becoming a diabetic or not. In fact, there are two times when weight control can actually prevent gestational diabetes and its future relative, adult-onset diabetes: *during pregnancy* and *in the postpartum*. Prevention is based on the threshold concept of how diabetes occurs. It is believed that everyone who has the genetic tendency to develop diabetes has a specific, although unknown, weight level at which diabetes is triggered. If you can stay under this weight, you can prevent— or at least postpone—the onset of diabetes. No army of psychic friends, no mountain-high pile of Ouija boards, nor any cave full of crystal balls can predict what this weight is—only you can!

Remember Karen? Let's take a closer look at what happened to her and you'll see what I mean. Karen weighed 165 pounds at 5'4" before conception. She never bothered to find out her risk factors for gestational diabetes because no one told her to. Now she knows better for the next pregnancy, and so do you. None of Karen's health care professionals told her that she was a sure bet for gestational diabetes. She herself had weighed 10 pounds at birth and was above 30 years of age when Justin was born. In addition, her father had diabetes, raising her odds. Unfortunately, she did not beat those odds. Later, she told me that had she known about the direct link between high weight gain during pregnancy and increased risk for gestational diabetes, she would have done her best to minimize the amount of weight she put on. Instead, she gained 55 pounds with Justin.

Let's suppose that Karen had known prior to becoming pregnant what she now knows about gestational diabetes and had decided to take a preventive approach. Instead of gaining 55 pounds, let's say she gained 45 pounds. This seemingly modest change would have had a major impact because it would have reduced her weight at delivery by about 10 pounds. Approximately 5 of those 10 pounds are fat! Keeping off those 5 pounds may have been enough to keep her body weight below her threshold weight for diabetes. In this way, by following some of the guidelines in Chapter Nine, Karen might have been able to avoid gestational diabetes.

Because the threshold for each person is unknown (until you get diabetes!), the first step in dealing with this issue is to know whether you have any of the risk factors for gestational diabetes. Review the list on page 177. If you have one or more of these risk factors, especially if you were overweight prior to conception, your index of suspicion should be high. If you have multiple risk factors, you should be on full gestational diabetes alert. You, like Karen, must keep your pregnancy weight to a minimum. Each pound that you avoid putting on during pregnancy can keep you below your diabetes threshold. Be sure to review the suggestions we made in Chapter Nine, to limit your pregnancy weight gain. I know that everyone and his mother are trying to force-feed you during your pregnancy. I know that everyone thinks it's okay for you to gain and gain because you're "eating for two"—but do you really need two diabetics? Minimizing your pregnancy weight gain to prevent gestational diabetes is just as important to the health of your baby as quitting smoking—and we all know the importance of that!

The fight against diabetes continues after delivery. Many health care professionals and books about postpartum health are quick to point out that gestational diabetes goes away when you deliver. They are right, but only *half* right. While the gestational diabetes itself goes away with the birth of your baby, the risk for developing adult-onset diabetes later in life does not. The biochemical cascade set in motion with your pregnancy can continue unnoticed. Like the corrosion in your home's plumbing, you are unaware of a problem until a pipe bursts. Diabetes can cause problems by blocking the small blood vessels of the heart, brain, and kidneys. Your blood test may show normal levels of glucose while damage is being done to your body's tiny blood vessels. You don't feel anything, and you have no symptoms until it's too late. However, those of you who had gestational diabetes have been forewarned. Therefore, you need to begin your weight loss efforts immediately after childbirth by following the three-trimester weight loss plan outlined in this book. This plan will work for those of you who had gestational diabetes, providing you don't require further insulin treatment. Those of you who do need insulin to control your sugar problems should see an endocrinologist, who is a medical doctor specializing in treating diabetes. The insulin-dependent diabetic has special needs regarding the timing of meals, total calories allowed, breast-feeding, and amount of carbohydrates and fats allowed. These needs can only be managed by a one-to-one relationship with a specialist, and the weight loss plan in this book may not by itself be suitable for you. However, our basic approach—limiting the amount of total fat consumed, increasing consumption of complex carbohydrates, and getting daily exercise—is the cornerstone for treating all forms of diabetes.

If you had gestational diabetes, you should be retested six weeks postpartum and at least once a year after that. While your doctor may make modifications to these recommendations, remember monitoring your health is *your* responsibility, too. By following the weight loss plan in this book, you are going to lose weight after delivery. But in order to keep diabetes at bay, you must be vigilant every day. You have a great head start; now keep it going! Postpartum weight loss by itself cuts your risk for future abnormal sugar problems in half! Daily exercise such as walking reduces your risk of diabetes by one-third! Just imagine the benefits of combining the two. Gestational diabetes is behind you; now, don't fall victim to its cousin—adult-onset diabetes. Act now and continue the sweet life—without the sugar!

Part IV

The Hello, Baby!
Good-bye, Baby Fat!
Eating Plan

Fourteen Days of Daily Menus

Daily Menu Day 1

Breakfast
1 whole wheat English muffin
1 teaspoon butter
1 egg, cooked as desired
1 cup skim milk

Snack
1 granola bar
½ cup skim milk
Nursing moms add 1 medium apple

Lunch
Pasta primavera:
• 1 cup cooked spinach pasta
• ½ cup Healthy Choice primavera sauce
5 Real Torino Classical Thin bread sticks
garden salad
2 tablespoons low-fat dressing

Snack
Jolly Time Light Microwave Popcorn,
4 cups popped
Nursing moms add 1 cup skim milk

Dinner
4-ounce tuna steak
1 cup pasta, cooked
½ cup Healthy Choice pasta sauce
1 cup brussels sprouts
Nursing moms add dinner roll and 1 teaspoon margarine

Snack
½ cup TCBY vanilla frozen yogurt
1 piece Sunshine Golden Fruit (cookie)

TOTAL CALORIES: 1590
% CALORIES FROM CARBOHYDRATES: 59
% CALORIES FROM FAT: 20
% CALORIES FROM PROTEIN: 21
Nursing moms add 320 calories

Postpartum Companion Page . . . Day 1

FOOD TIPS . . .
- When you have that chocolate craving, try low-fat chocolate pudding or hot cocoa.
- Opt for brown rice over white rice. . . . Brown rice contains 10 percent rice bran, which has been shown to lower cholesterol.
- Make your own ground chicken or turkey (ask your butcher to grind it for you). . . . The commercial kind includes fatty skin.

LIFESTYLE TIPS . . .
- Eat in the kitchen or dining room. All other rooms should be out of bounds for eating.
- Freeze leftovers so they won't be handy for nibbling.

DID YOU KNOW . . .
- Carnival Cruise's "Fun Ships" (twelve in all) serve eight meals and snacks every day of their vacations at sea. Some of the eye-popping consumption totals for the fleet each week include:

  56,800 pounds of chicken
  393,660 eggs
  328,000 bacon slices
  13,500 pounds of pasta
  250,800 cans of soft drinks
  42,420 bottles of wine

INSTANT INSPIRATION . . .

"The secret of getting ahead is getting started."
—Sally Berger

"If you focus on results, you will never change. If you focus on change, you will get results."
—Jack Dixon

Daily Menu Day 2

Breakfast

1 large whole wheat bagel
2 tablespoons Philadelphia Light cream cheese
½ cup skim milk
Nursing moms have 1 cup skim milk

Snack

1 medium orange
**Nursing moms add 1 slice whole wheat toast and 1 tablespoon peanut
butter**

Lunch

1 Morningstar Farms Garden Veggie Patty
1 slice cheese
1 hamburger roll
garden salad
2 tablespoons low-fat/nonfat dressing
½ cup skim milk

Snack

1½ ounces Baked Tostitos tortilla chips
2 tablespoons nacho cheese dip

Dinner

1 serving Chicken Marsala (see recipe, page 218)
1 cup cooked brown rice
1 cup cooked broccoli

Snack

1 Weight Watchers Gourmet Apple Cinnamon muffin
½ cup skim milk
Nursing moms have 1 cup skim milk

TOTAL CALORIES: 1655
% CALORIES FROM CARBOHYDRATES: 58
% CALORIES FROM FAT: 18
% CALORIES FROM PROTEIN: 24
Nursing moms add 245 calories

Postpartum Companion Page . . . Day 2

FOOD TIPS . . .
- Use nonfat yogurt instead of sour cream.
- Use lemon juice and mustard as condiments instead of mayonnaise.
- Use applesauce, mashed bananas, or prune paste instead of shortening when baking.

LIFESTYLE TIPS . . .
- Switch the channel when a food commercial comes on.
- Sit up straight. . . . You burn 10 percent more calories sitting upright than reclining.

DID YOU KNOW . . .
- More children are born in September than any other month.
- Worldwide $10 billion per year is spent on pet food. . . . Worldwide, $7 billion annually is spent on baby food.
- A typical American child will have consumed 500 peanut butter and jelly sandwiches by high school.

INSTANT INSPIRATION . . .

"A solid fantasy can totally transform one million realities."

"See, you don't have to think about the right thing. If you are for the right thing, you do it without thinking."
—Maya Angelou

Daily Menu Day 3

Breakfast

1 cup plain oatmeal or ½ cup flavored

½ cup skim milk

1 medium orange

Snack

2 graham crackers (large)

½ cup skim milk

Nursing moms have 4 graham crackers

Lunch

Grilled chicken sandwich:

- roll
- chicken breast, 4 ounce
- lettuce/tomato
- 1 piece cheese
- 1 tablespoon light mayonnaise

½ cup skim milk

Snack

½ whole wheat bagel

2 teaspoons Philadelphia Light cream cheese, plain

1 tablespoon jelly

Nursing moms add 1 cup skim milk

Dinner

4 ounces lean London broil

1 cup green beans

1 cup mashed potatoes (with milk and margarine)

Snack

1 Snackwell's Low Fat Ice Cream Sandwich

Nursing moms have 1 cup low-fat frozen yogurt

TOTAL CALORIES: 1676

% CALORIES FROM CARBOHYDRATES: 50

% CALORIES FROM FAT: 25

% CALORIES FROM PROTEIN: 25

Nursing moms add 250 calories

Postpartum Companion Page . . . Day 3

FOOD TIPS . . .
- Margarine contains the same amount of fat as butter . . . so use it sparingly.
- A Lifesavers candy contains 10 calories, while a sugar-free breath mint contains 3 calories.
- Soybeans, pea beans, and black beans are the top flatulence producers.

LIFESTYLE TIPS . . .
- Put your fork down while you chew your food.
- Eat a light snack before going to a party where you may be tempted to overeat
- Take a nap when your baby naps.

DID YOU KNOW . . .
- The average American consumes 4000 calories on Thanksgiving Day.
- Approximately 95 percent of all babies are born in hospitals. The other 5 percent are born at home or on trains, planes, and buses.
- On an average day, 2,160,000 Hershey's Kisses are produced.

INSTANT INSPIRATION . . .

"To be a star you must shine your own light, follow your own path, and don't worry about the darkness, for that is when stars shine brightest."
—Unknown

"It is easy to halve the potato where there is love."
—Irish proverb

Daily Menu Day 4

Breakfast

2 frozen waffles

¼ cup low-calorie syrup

1 cup skim milk

Snack

1 medium apple

½ cup low-fat cottage cheese

Nursing moms add 2 tablespoons wheat germ and ½ cup skim milk

Lunch

3½ ounces spinach

1 chopped egg, hard-boiled

1 ounce Athenos crumbled feta cheese

1 tablespoon Bac* O's

2 tablespoons low-fat/nonfat salad dressing

1 whole wheat pita

½ cup skim milk

Snack

Nutri-Grain cereal bar

½ cup skim milk

Nursing moms have 1 cup skim milk and add 1 small banana

Dinner

1 serving Cheese Polenta with Spaghetti Sauce (see recipe, page 218)

2 slices Italian bread

garden salad

2 tablespoons low-fat/nonfat salad dressing

1 cup cooked green beans

Snack

2 large graham crackers

½ cup fruited yogurt, Dannon 99% fat free

Nursing moms add 1 cup skim milk

TOTAL CALORIES: 1710

% CALORIES FROM CARBOHYDRATES: 62

% CALORIES FROM FAT: 20

% CALORIES FROM PROTEIN: 18

Nursing moms add 295 calories

Postpartum Companion Page . . . Day 4

FOOD TIPS . . .
- Try not to chew gum. It will stimulate your appetite.
- Try mustard or salsa as a topping for your baked potato.
- Exposure to fluorescent light or to sunlight may result in a loss of vitamins and flavor in milk bought in clear plastic containers.

LIFESTYLE TIPS . . .
- Eating on small plates teaches portion control.
- Standing while talking on the telephone burns an extra 3 calories per minute.

DID YOU KNOW . . .
- There are 500,000 more unmarried couples living together now than in 1970.
- Americans eat an average of 11 pounds of peanuts per year and one-fourth of the peanuts grown end up in candy.
- The most popular green vegetable is broccoli.

INSTANT INSPIRATION . . .

"One can never consent to creep when one feels an impulse to soar."

"Alone we can do so little, together we can do so much."

"Life is a daring adventure or nothing at all."
—Helen Keller

Daily Menu Day 5

Breakfast

1 cup cornflakes/Product 19/Total

1 cup skim milk

1 small banana

1 slice raisin toast

½ teaspoon margarine

Snack

1 cup Dannon low-fat fruited yogurt

Nursing moms add 1 cup skim milk

Lunch

Tuna on a bagel:

- ½ can tuna packed in water
- 1 tablespoon light mayonnaise
- 1 whole wheat bagel

1 cup skim milk

Snack

Entenmann's Light Golden Loaf, 1 serving

½ cup skim milk

Dinner

1 serving Chicken Stroganoff (see recipe, page 221)

garden salad

½ cup egg noodles, cooked

1 teaspoon butter

Nursing moms have 1 cup egg noodles

Snack

4-ounce cup Swiss Miss Fat-Free pudding snack

Nursing moms add 6 gingersnaps

TOTAL CALORIES: 1792

% CALORIES FROM CARBOHYDRATES: 60

% CALORIES FROM FAT: 18

% CALORIES FROM PROTEIN: 22

Nursing moms add 320 calories

Postpartum Companion Page . . . Day 5

FOOD TIPS

- Häagen-Dazs super premium-type ice cream contains nearly twice the fat of a regular ice cream like Edy's Grand.
- Dark meat chicken contains twice the fat of white meat chicken.
- A carrot stick contains 5 calories. A celery stick contains 6 calories.

LIFESTYLE TIPS . . .

- Park at the furthest end of the shopping mall.
- Try interval strolling: speed up for 30 seconds and then slow down for 30 seconds. . . . Continue until you've reached your destination.

DID YOU KNOW . . .

- One-third of the ice cream sold is vanilla.
- Walking is the most popular exercise in the United States.
- The average American female is a size 14.

INSTANT INSPIRATION . . .

"I am not afraid of storms, for I'm learning how to sail my ship."
—Louisa May Alcott

"Nothing is worth more than this day."
—Goethe

Daily Menu Day 6

Breakfast

2 slices French toast:
- 2 slices white bread
- 2 eggs
- 1 tsp margarine

¼ cup low calorie syrup

½ cup skim milk

Snack

1 small banana

Nursing moms add 1 cup low-fat cottage cheese

Lunch

Lean roast beef or turkey sandwich:
- 1 whole wheat pita bread
- 3 slices lean roast beef or turkey
- 1 tablespoon light mayonnaise

½ cup skim milk

Snack

1 Jell-O Gelatin snack

Nursing moms add 1 cup skim milk

Dinner

4 ounces salmon, broiled

1 large baked potato and skin

2 tablespoons sour cream

½ cup cooked broccoli

Snack

1½-ounce bag thin pretzels

½ cup skim milk

Nursing moms have 1 cup skim milk

TOTAL CALORIES: 1610

% CALORIES FROM CARBOHYDRATES: 54

% CALORIES FROM FAT: 23

% CALORIES FROM PROTEIN: 23

Nursing moms add 280 calories

Postpartum Companion Page . . . Day 6

FOOD TIPS . . .
- Hot dishes tend to fill you up faster than cold ones.
- Try whole wheat pasta instead of regular pasta. . . . The former contains close to four times as much fiber as the latter.
- There are ten teaspoons of sugar in one can of Coca-Cola. . . . Get used to the taste of seltzer or iced tea, or rediscover water!

LIFESTYLE TIPS . . .
- Stay out of the kitchen between meals.
- Always go shopping with a food list.

DID YOU KNOW . . .
- The average child laughs 300 times per day and the average adult laughs between 50 and 100 times per day.
- Your weight is different at different times of the day. You weigh the least at 7:00 A.M. and the most at 6:00 P.M.
- Regular ground turkey and regular ground beef have equivalent amounts of fat.

INSTANT INSPIRATION . . .

"Keep your face always toward the sunshine and the shadows will fall behind you."
—Unknown

"Success is measured not so much by the position that one has reached in life as by the obstacles which he has overcome while trying to succeed."
—Booker T. Washington

Daily Menu Day 7

Breakfast

1 whole wheat English muffin

1 teaspoon margarine

2 eggs, cooked as desired

½ cup skim milk

Snack

1 Snackwell's Hearty Fruit 'n' Grain Bar

½ cup skim milk

Nursing moms add small banana

Lunch

Empire Kosher turkey frank

Arnold hot dog bun

½ cup vegetarian baked beans

garden salad

2 tablespoons low-fat/nonfat dressing

Snack

1 cup low-fat frozen yogurt

Nursing moms add 1 cup skim milk and 2 tablespoons wheat germ

Dinner

1 cup cooked pasta

½ cup Healthy Choice marinara sauce

1 small ear of corn

2 small slices Italian bread

1 teaspoon butter

Snack

2 Mother's multigrain rice cakes

½ cup skim milk

Nursing moms have 1 cup skim milk

TOTAL CALORIES: 1727

% CALORIES FROM CARBOHYDRATES: 60

% CALORIES FROM FAT: 22

% CALORIES FROM PROTEIN: 18

Nursing moms add 250 calories

Postpartum Companion Page . . . Day 7

FOOD TIPS . . .
- Nonfat pretzels contain the same amount of fat as regular pretzels.
- The brown breads (multigrain, whole wheat, etc.) are generally more nutritious than white bread, but check the ingredients because some brands contain caramelized sugar and other ingredients to enhance color and taste.
- A pink grapefruit is pink because it contains 27 times more beta carotene than a white grapefruit.

LIFESTYLE TIPS . . .
- Eat cereal for dinner occasionally.
- Exercise in the evening after you have eaten dinner because exercise stimulates your appetite.

DID YOU KNOW . . .
- America's favorite breakfast is cold cereal.
- Over the past ten years, the average American adult has gained 8 pounds.
- Asparagus contains sulfur, which can make your urine smell.

INSTANT INSPIRATION . . .

"The future belongs to those who believe in the beauty of their dream."

"You must do everything you think you cannot do."

"No one can make you feel inferior without your consent."
—Eleanor Roosevelt

Daily Menu Day 8

Breakfast

1 cup plain oatmeal or ½ cup flavored

½ cup skim milk

1 medium orange

Snack

½ whole wheat bagel

½ cup low-fat cottage cheese

tomato slice

½ cup skim milk

Nursing moms have 1 cup skim milk and add 1 small banana

Lunch

1 serving Chicken Chestnut Salad (see recipe, page 223)

1 dinner roll (hard roll)

½ cup low-fat frozen yogurt

Snack

Kudos chocolate chip granola bar

½ cup skim milk

Dinner

4 ounces broiled swordfish

1 cup cooked brown rice

1 cup cooked green beans

1 teaspoon margarine

½ cup skim milk

Snack

1 cup fruit cocktail in water

Nursing moms add 1 cup skim milk and ½ cup low-fat fruited yogurt

TOTAL CALORIES: 1630

% CALORIES FROM CARBOHYDRATES: 59

% CALORIES FROM FAT: 18

% CALORIES FROM PROTEIN: 23

Nursing moms add 235 calories

Postpartum Companion Page . . . Day 8

FOOD TIPS . . .
- Beans are an excellent source of protein and are low in fat. A cup of cooked kidney beans supplies 16 grams of protein and 0.9 gram of fat.
- Skim milk has less fat than whole milk; it contains slightly more calcium, as well.
- Olives get 85 percent of their calories from fat and are very high in sodium.

LIFESTYLE TIPS . . .
- Never go food shopping on an empty stomach.
- Drink water or seltzer 15 minutes before a meal. . . . It will fill you up.

DID YOU KNOW . . .
- The average American eats about 15 pounds of beans per year, and consumption is increasing.
- The average baby eats 880 jars of baby food in the first 18 months of life.
- Over a lifetime, taste outlasts all other senses.

INSTANT INSPIRATION . . .

"We are what we repeatedly do, excellence is therefore not an act but a habit."
—Aristotle

"Impossible is a word only to be found in the dictionary of fools."
—Napoleon

Daily Menu Day 9

Breakfast

1 whole wheat English muffin
1½ tablespoon jelly
2 tablespoons Philadelphia Light cream cheese
½ cup skim milk

Snack

1 medium orange
Nursing moms add 1 cup low-fat fruited yogurt, Dannon

Lunch

Mozzarella and tomato salad:
- 2½ ounces part-skim mozzarella
- sliced fresh tomato
- 2 tablespoons balsamic vinegar
- ½ Toufayan pita bread

½ cup skim milk

Snack

1½ ounces Baked Tostitos tortilla chips
3 tablespoons black bean dip

Dinner

1 serving Oregano-Garlic Chicken Breasts (see recipe, page 219)
1 cup cooked pasta
½ cup cooked spinach
Nursing moms add 1 cup skim milk and 1 dinner roll with 1 teaspoon margarine

Snack

1 Snackwell's Low Fat Ice Cream Sandwich

TOTAL CALORIES: 1648
% CALORIES FROM CARBOHYDRATES: 55
% CALORIES FROM FAT: 22
% CALORIES FROM PROTEIN: 23
Nursing moms add 346 calories

Postpartum Companion Page . . . Day 9

FOOD TIPS . . .
- Shrimp is very low in fat but high in cholesterol. A 3-ounce portion has 1 gram of fat, but can contain 130 milligrams of cholesterol.
- Three ounces of tuna fish in oil contains 7 fat grams, while 3 ounces of tuna in water contains 2 fat grams.
- Even though lobsters are rich in taste, they are relatively low in fat and cholesterol.

LIFESTYLE TIPS . . .
- When in a restaurant, ask for salad dressing on the side and your entree's gravy or sauce on the side as well.
- When dining out, look for terms like baked, broiled, steamed, poached, lightly sautéed, or stir-fried.

DID YOU KNOW . . .
- The three most popular American fruits are bananas, apples, and seedless grapes.
- The average American makes 3½ pounds of garbage a day.
- We throw away 60 million pounds of food a day.

INSTANT INSPIRATION . . .

"Babies come into the world holding joy in their hands. And when they open those small fingers, the whole world's supply is replenished, again."
—Unknown

"Success is a journey, not a destination."
—Ben Sweetland

Daily Menu Day 10

Breakfast

1½ cups Cheerios

1 cup skim milk

1 small banana

Snack

JJ Flats breadflats, 2 pieces

½ cup skim milk

Nursing moms have 1 cup skim milk

Lunch

Turkey breast sandwich on bagel:

- bagel
- 3 slices lean turkey
- lettuce/tomato
- 1 tablespoon low-fat mayonnaise

Snack

Hendrie's frozen fudge stick

Nursing moms add 1 cup skim milk

Dinner

1 serving Chinese Flank Steak (see recipe, page 220)

½ cup cooked rice

½ cup cooked broccoli

Nursing moms have 1 cup rice and add 1 cup skim milk

Snack

Jolly Time Light Microwave Popcorn,

4 cups popped

½ cup skim milk

TOTAL CALORIES: 1530

% CALORIES FROM CARBOHYDRATES: 53

% CALORIES FROM FAT: 24

% CALORIES FROM PROTEIN: 23

Nursing moms add 300 calories

Postpartum Companion Page . . . Day 10

FOOD TIPS . . .
- Try unsweetened cereals and those containing fiber for breakfast— fiber is good for the entire family!
- Go salsa! Two tablespoons of butter on a baked potato add an extra 200 calories and 22 grams of fat. One-fourth cup of salsa adds only 18 calories and no fat.
- Avoid the healthy sound of carrot cake. Very often it has double the calories of the "guilty-sounding" chocolate cake.

LIFESTYLE TIPS . . .
- Concentrate on eating. When you eat while reading or watching T.V., you can easily overeat.
- If you wish to reduce your portion size while dining out, order an appetizer as your entrée.

DID YOU KNOW . . .
- The average adult's skin weighs approximately ten pounds.
- Fats tend to float to the top of watery stomach contents, which is why high-fat foods make us feel full.
- Your brain's internal clock slows as you age, altering your sense of time and making it seem to pass more quickly.

INSTANT INSPIRATION . . .

"Joy is not in things; it is in us."
—Wagner

"Scientists have proven that it is impossible to long-jump thirty feet. But I don't listen to that kind of talk. Thoughts like that have a way of sinking into your feet."
—Carl Lewis

Daily Menu Day 11

Breakfast
2 whole grain frozen waffles
¼ cup light syrup
1 cup skim milk

Snack
1 small banana
Nursing moms add 1 cup skim milk and 2 graham crackers

Lunch
Peanut butter and jelly sandwich:
- 1½ tablespoons peanut butter
- 1½ tablespoons jelly
- 2 slices whole wheat bread

½ cup skim milk

Snack
1 Jell-O pudding snack
½ cup skim milk

Dinner
1 serving Chicken Cacciatore (see recipe, page 221)
¾ cup cooked pasta
Nursing moms add a dinner roll and 1 tablespoon margarine

Snack
½ whole wheat bagel
1 tablespoon jelly
1 tablespoon cream cheese
Nursing moms add 1 cup skim milk

TOTAL CALORIES: 1715
% CALORIES FROM CARBOHYDRATES: 59
% CALORIES FROM FAT: 22
% CALORIES FROM PROTEIN: 19
Nursing moms add 326 calories

Postpartum Companion Page . . . Day 11

FOOD TIPS
- Include plenty of soybeans and tofu in your diet. . . . They have been shown to lower the risk of breast cancer.
- Watch the tuna salad in a restaurant. . . . A B.L.T. has fewer calories and fat than a tuna salad sandwich.
- When making an omelet, try using the whites only for all but one egg. . . . You will forgo much of the fat and cholesterol.

LIFESTYLE TIPS . . .
- Avoid buffet-style meals because portion control is nearly impossible.
- Opt for the stairs versus the elevator when baby is not in tow

DID YOU KNOW . . .
- America's favorite pizza topping is pepperoni, whereas in Poland the favorite toppings on a Domino's pizza are cabbage and sausage.
- A zinc deficiency can cause acne, hair loss, and male impotence.
- Breakfast eaters have a metabolic rate 4 to 5 percent higher than non-breakfast eaters.

INSTANT INSPIRATION . . .

"You don't stop laughing because you grow old, you grow old because you stop laughing."
—Michael Pritchard

"You may have to fight battles more than once to win it."
—Margaret Thatcher

Daily Menu Day 12

Breakfast

1 cup plain oatmeal, or ½ cup flavored

1 cup skim milk

1 medium orange

Nursing moms add ½ oat bran English muffin and 1 teaspoon margarine

Snack

1 small banana

2 Mother's multigrain rice cakes

1 tablespoon jelly

Lunch

Lean roast beef or turkey sandwich:

• 2 slices whole wheat bread

• 3 slices lean roast beef or turkey

• 1 tablespoon mayonnaise

½ cup skim milk

Nursing moms add ½ cup skim milk

Snack

Weight Watchers Smart Ones vanilla ice cream sandwich

Dinner

2 slices Pizza Hut Thin 'n' Crispy cheese pizza (medium pie)

garden salad

2 tablespoons Marie's Fat Free Red Wine Vinaigrette dressing

1 cup skim milk

Snack

1 cup Colombo low-fat fruited yogurt

Nursing moms add 2 tablespoons wheat germ and ½ cup skim milk

TOTAL CALORIES: 1570

% CALORIES FROM CARBOHYDRATES: 57

% CALORIES FROM FAT: 22

% CALORIES FROM PROTEIN: 21

Nursing moms add 270 calories

Postpartum Companion Page . . . Day 12

FOOD TIPS . . .
- Purple grape juice may lower heart attack risk as much as aspirin.
- Choose Florida avocados over California ones; they're lower in calories and sodium.
- Choose American grapes over European grapes; they contain nearly half the calories.

LIFESTYLE TIPS . . .
- Grab support anywhere you can.
- Transfer your oil and vinegar dressing to a spray bottle, and you will use less.

DID YOU KNOW . . .
- The snacking industry is a $15 billion per year industry. Potato chips account for $3 billion.
- Lovemaking can burn between 150 and 300 calories per session . . . depending on the fervor.
- Americans drink approximately 2.7 billion gallons of bottled water per year.

INSTANT INSPIRATION . . .

"Kind words can be short and easy to speak, but their echoes are truly endless."

"We can do no great things, only small things with great love."
—Mother Teresa

Daily Menu Day 13

Breakfast
1 whole wheat English muffin
1 teaspoon margarine
2 eggs (if fried, use nonstick spray)
1 cup skim milk

Snack
1 medium apple
Nursing moms add 2 tablespoon peanut butter and 1 cup skim milk

Lunch
Tuna sandwich:
- ½ can tuna packed in water
- 1 tablespoon light mayonnaise
- 2 slices rye or whole wheat bread

1 cup of skim milk

Snack
1 Quaker Low Fat Chewy Granola Bar

Dinner
1 cup cooked spaghetti
½ cup Healthy Choice brand marinara sauce
2 small slices Italian bread
1 teaspoon margarine
garden salad
2 tablespoons Good Seasons Fat Free Creamy Italian salad dressing

Snack
1 cup TCBY Dutch chocolate low-fat frozen yogurt
Nursing moms add 1 cup skim milk

TOTAL CALORIES: 1680
% CALORIES FROM CARBOHYDRATES: 54
% CALORIES FROM FAT: 26
% CALORIES FROM PROTEIN: 20
Nursing moms add 350 calories

Postpartum Companion Page . . . Day 13

FOOD TIPS . . .

- Replace your morning orange juice with prune juice. The latter helps prevent constipation, which is especially a problem for those new mothers who have had an episiotomy.
- When at the movies consider this: A medium-sized tub of popcorn contains 650 calories, of which 300 are fat calories.
- Sprinkle-on margarine powders are made from carbohydrates and contain little or no fat. These powders will melt on potatoes and other hot foods; however, they are not spreadable.

LIFESTYLE TIPS . . .

- Portion control can be facilitated by eating a meal with chopsticks or with a cocktail fork.
- Even if you don't smoke, secondhand smoke is harmful to a fetus, newborn, or child.

DID YOU KNOW . . .

- A study shows that women who eat tomato sauce twice a week have a lower risk of developing asthma. Tomatoes also contain lycopene, a powerful antioxidant that helps prevent lung and colon cancer.
- Fifteen million Americans have adult-onset diabetes, and 7 million don't even know that they have it.
- A typical airline lunch or dinner contains 800 calories.

INSTANT INSPIRATION . . .

"To be successful, you don't have to do extraordinary things. Just do ordinary things extraordinarily well."
—John Rohn

"Plenty of people miss their share of happiness, not because they never found it, but because they didn't stop to enjoy it."
—William Feather

Daily Menu Day 14

Breakfast

1 cup of cornflakes/Product 19/Total

1 cup skim milk

1 small banana

Snack

1 cup low-fat fruit/yogurt

Nursing moms add 2 tablespoons wheat germ

Lunch

Pita with melted cheese and tomato:

- 1 whole wheat pita bread
- 2 slices Swiss cheese
- 3 slices fresh tomato

½ cup skim milk

Snack

½ cup lemon sorbet

2 tablespoons wheat germ

Nursing moms add 2 large graham crackers and 1 cup skim milk

Dinner

1 serving Lemon Chicken with Thyme (see recipe, page 222)

¾ cup cooked brown rice

½ cup cooked broccoli

½ cup skim milk

Snack

2 Pepperidge Farm Fruitful raspberry tart cookies

½ cup skim milk

Nursing moms have 1 cup skim milk

TOTAL CALORIES: 1640

% CALORIES FROM CARBOHYDRATES: 54

% CALORIES FROM FAT: 24

% CALORIES FROM PROTEIN: 22

Nursing moms add 290 calories

Postpartum Companion Page . . . Day 14

FOOD TIPS . . .
- One cup of taco salad contains 300 calories, of which 200 are fat calories.
- Ounce for ounce, kiwi fruits have more vitamin C than oranges, as much potassium as bananas, more vitamin E than avocados, and more dietary fiber than most cereals . . . and they contain only 45 calories per fruit!
- Hot spicy foods have been shown to curb appetite in scientific studies.

LIFESTYLE TIPS . . .
- Brushing and flossing immediately after dinner will discourage late-night snacking.
- At parties, do not plant yourself near the food.

DID YOU KNOW . . .
- A woman born in 1900 had a life expectancy of 47 years.
- A woman born in 1988 has a life expectancy of 75 years.
- A woman born in 1998 has a life expectancy of 82 years, 6 years more than a man.

INSTANT INSPIRATION . . .

"If we don't change direction soon, we'll end up where we are going."
—Professor Irwin Corey

"Failure is the opportunity to intelligently begin again."
—Henry Ford

Recipes

Chicken Marsala

4-ounce skinless, boneless chicken
   breasts
¼ cup Egg Beaters or egg whites
½ cup crushed wheat crackers
1 teaspoon minced garlic

2 tablespoons chicken broth
¼ cup marsala wine or red wine
1 chicken bouillon cube
dash of ground pepper
2 tablespoons chopped parsley

Pound the chicken breasts to a ¼-inch thickness. Dip in the Egg Beaters or egg whites and then coat with the crushed crackers. Set aside.

In a nonstick skillet, cook the minced garlic in the broth for 1 to 2 minutes. Add the chicken, and cook for approximately 6 minutes, turning once. Remove to a serving platter; keep warm.

In the same skillet, add the wine, bouillon cube, pepper, and parsley. Cook and stir until the mixture thickens and begins to boil. If it is too dry, add 1 to 3 tablespoons broth. Spoon over the chicken and serve.

MAKES 4 SERVINGS

NUTRITIONAL VALUES PER 4-OUNCE SERVING: calories—191, protein—28 grams, fat—6 grams, carbohydrates—6 grams

Cheese Polenta with Spaghetti Sauce

1 cup cornmeal
several drops of hot pepper sauce
¼ cup grated Parmesan cheese

1 cup shredded low-fat mozzarella
⅔ cup chopped red bell pepper
1 cup low-fat spaghetti sauce

In a large saucepan, bring 2⅔ cups of water to a boil. In a bowl, combine the cornmeal and hot pepper sauce with 1 cup cold water. Add the mixture to boiling water, stirring continuously. Cook until the mixture comes to a boil. Reduce heat and simmer for another 10 to 15 minutes until the mixture is thick, stirring often.

Pour and spread half the mixture in a 9-inch pie plate. Cover with 2 tablespoons Parmesan cheese, the mozzarella cheese, and the chopped pepper. Add the remaining half of the cornmeal mixture and the remaining Parmesan cheese. Cover and refrigerate several hours until firm.

Bake, uncovered, at 400 degrees for 30 to 35 minutes.

MAKES 4 SERVINGS
NUTRITIONAL VALUES PER SERVING: calories—251, fat—7 grams, protein—14 grams, carbohydrates—16 grams

Oregano-Garlic Chicken Breasts

¼ cup lemon juice

5 cloves garlic, minced or crushed

1 teaspoon oregano

¼ teaspoon pepper

four 4-ounce skinless, boneless
   chicken breasts

1 medium onion

¼ cup cornstarch

1 tablespoon margarine

1 tablespoon olive oil

¾ cup chicken broth

¼ cup minced fresh chives or
   scallion greens

2½ tablespoons grated lemon zest

pinch of sugar

In a shallow 11- × 17-inch baking dish, combine the lemon juice, the garlic, ¾ teaspoon oregano, and the pepper. Add the chicken, turn to coat well with the seasonings, and set aside to marinate for 10 minutes.

Cut the onion into thin wedges. Place the cornstarch on a plate or in a shallow bowl.

Remove the chicken from the marinade, reserving the marinade. Dredge the chicken lightly in the cornstarch; reserve the excess cornstarch.

In a large skillet, warm the margarine in the olive oil over medium-high heat until the margarine is melted. Place the chicken in the skillet and cook for 5 minutes on each side. Remove the chicken to a plate and cover loosely to keep warm.

Add the onion to the skillet and stir-fry until it begins to soften, 1 to 2 minutes. In a small bowl, blend the chicken broth with the reserved cornstarch. Add the broth mixture, reserved marinade, remaining ¼ teaspoon oregano, 2 tablespoons chives, lemon zest, and sugar to the skillet, and bring to a boil.

continued

Return the chicken (and any juices that have accumulated on the plate) to the skillet and cook for 2 to 3 minutes, or until the chicken is cooked through.

Serve the chicken topped with the onion and sauce and sprinkle with the remaining 2 tablespoons chives.

MAKES 4 SERVINGS
NUTRITIONAL VALUES PER SERVING: calories—265, protein—34 grams, fat—8 grams, carbohydrates—12 grams

Chinese Flank Steak and Low-Fat "Not-Fried Rice"

1½ pounds lean flank steak

MARINADE:
2 tablespoons low-sodium soy sauce
2 teaspoons honey
¼ cup cider vinegar
¼ teaspoon tabasco sauce

Place the flank steak in a shallow dish. In a bowl, combine the marinade ingredients and mix well. Pour over the flank steak. Cover and refrigerate for 24 hours. When ready to cook, remove the flank steak from the marinade and broil or grill. Serve with "Not-Fried Rice."

RICE
PAM spray
½ cup finely chopped onion
2 cups plus 1 tablespoon chicken broth
1 tablespoon sherry or cooking sherry
1 tablespoon low-sodium soy sauce
4 drops Tabasco sauce
1 cup uncooked long-grain converted rice
⅓ cup diagonally sliced green onions
1 tablespoon toasted pine nuts

Coat a medium saucepan with PAM spray. Place over medium heat until hot. Add onion and sauté in 1 tablespoon chicken broth for about 2 minutes. Add 2 cups chicken broth and the sherry, soy sauce, and Tabasco sauce and bring to a boil. Stir in rice, cover, reduce the heat and simmer for 25 minutes or until the rice is tender and the liquid is absorbed. Remove from the heat and stir in the green onions and pine nuts.

MAKES 6 SERVINGS
NUTRITIONAL VALUES PER 4-OUNCE SERVING OF STEAK AND ½ CUP RICE: calories—327, protein—22 grams, fat—12 grams, carbohydrates—31 grams

Chicken Cacciatore

2 tablespoons chicken broth
six 4-ounce skinless, boneless
    chicken breasts
1 chopped onion
2 teaspoons minced garlic
1 cup tomato sauce
one 16-ounce can Italian tomatoes

½ cup white wine
¼ teaspoon basil
¼ teaspoon oregano
1 bay leaf
½ teaspoon salt
1 cup sliced mushrooms
pasta

Heat the chicken broth in a nonstick skillet and brown the chicken, onion, and garlic. Add all the other ingredients except the mushrooms and pasta. Bring to a boil, then cover and simmer for 30 minutes. Add the mushrooms and cook for 10 minutes more. Remove the chicken from the skillet and boil down the sauce until slightly thickened. Serve with pasta.

MAKES 6 SERVINGS
NUTRITIONAL VALUES PER 4-OUNCE SERVING OF CHICKEN: calories—217, protein—30 grams, fat—3.5 grams, carbohydrates—17 grams

Chicken Stroganoff

four 4-ounce chicken breasts
¼ teaspoon garlic powder
¼ teaspoon white pepper
½ cup low-fat cream of mushroom
    soup

1 cup plain yogurt
one 6-ounce can sliced mushrooms,
    drained
2 tablespoons sherry
¼ cup Parmesan cheese

Preheat oven to 350 degrees.

Spray on 8- ×11-inch casserole dish with nonstick cooking spray. Place chicken breasts in casserole dish. Do not overlap. Sprinkle with garlic and pepper. Combine soup, yogurt, and mushrooms and pour over chicken. Sprinkle cheese over all. Bake for 30 minutes or microwave on high, covered for 18 minutes or until chicken is tender. Serve with noodles.

NUTRITIONAL VALUES PER 4-OUNCE SERVING OF CHICKEN: calories—202, protein—28 grams, fat—6 grams, carbohydrates—15 grams

Lemon Chicken with Thyme

3 tablespoons flour
½ teaspoon salt
¼ teaspoon pepper
four 4-ounce skinless, boneless
   chicken breasts
2 tablespoons olive oil
1 medium onion

1 tablespoon margarine
1 cup chicken broth
3 tablespoons lemon juice
½ teaspoon thyme
lemon wedges and 2 tablespoons
   chopped parsley (optional)

In a plastic bag, combine the flour, salt, and pepper, and shake to mix. Add the chicken and shake to coat lightly. Remove the chicken and reserve the excess seasoned flour.

In a large skillet, warm 1 tablespoon olive oil over medium heat. Add the chicken and brown on one side, about 5 minutes. Add the remaining tablespoon olive oil, turn the chicken, and brown well on the second side, about 5 minutes longer. Transfer the chicken to a plate and set aside.

Coarsely chop the onion. Add the margarine to the skillet. When the margarine melts, add the onion and cook, stirring, until softened, 2 to 3 minutes.

Stir in the reserved seasoned flour and cook, stirring, until the flour is completely incorporated, about 1 minute.

Add the broth, 2 tablespoons lemon juice, and the thyme, and bring the mixture to a boil, stirring constantly.

Return the chicken to the skillet, reduce the heat to medium-low, and cover. Cook until the chicken is tender and opaque, about 5 minutes.

Divide the chicken among 4 plates. Stir the remaining 1 tablespoon lemon juice into the sauce in the skillet and pour over the chicken. Garnish the chicken with lemon wedges and sprinkled parsley, if desired.

MAKES 4 SERVINGS
NUTRITIONAL VALUES PER SERVING: calories—250, protein—28 grams, fat—12 grams, carbohydrates—7 grams

Chicken Chestnut Salad

3 cups shredded romaine lettuce
1 whole chicken breast, boiled,
   boned, and sliced
1 cup carrots, julienned
2 scallions, shredded
½ cup chopped chestnuts, steamed
   or boiled

DRESSING
1 tablespoon wine vinegar
2 tablespoons sesame oil
1 teaspoon reduced-sodium soy
   sauce
1 teaspoon hoisin sauce
1 teaspoon finely minced ginger
1 teaspoon sugar
1 teaspoon hot chili oil

Put the salad ingredients in a bowl. Mix the dressing ingredients in another bowl, then toss with the salad.

MAKES 4 SERVINGS
NUTRITIONAL VALUES PER SERVING: calories—162, protein—12 grams, fat—4 grams, carbohydrates—20 grams

Bran Muffins with Dried Fruit

1 cup flour
1½ teaspoons baking powder
1½ teaspoons baking soda
½ teaspoon cinnamon
2 cups bran cereal
1½ cups low-fat milk

⅓ cup firmly packed brown sugar
1 egg
½ cup applesauce
½ cup dried apricots, julienned
½ cup currants or raisins

Preheat the oven to 400 degrees.

In a bowl mix the flour, baking soda, baking powder, and cinnamon.

In another bowl, mix the cereal, milk, brown sugar, and egg. Let stand for 5 minutes, and then stir in the applesauce, apricots, and currants.

Add the dry ingredients to the mixture.

Spoon the mixture into a nonstick 12-muffin pan and bake for 18 to 20 minutes.

MAKES 12 SERVINGS

NUTRITIONAL VALUES PER SERVING: calories—173, protein—4 grams, fat—1 gram, carbohydrates—32 grams

Lemon Chicken Noodle Soup

7 cups low-sodium canned chicken broth

6 cloves garlic, minced

½ cup diced tiny carrots

2 parsnips, peeled and diced

2 celery ribs, diced

2 onions

3 tablespoons fresh lemon juice

1½ cups dry broad egg noodles

1 skinless, boneless chicken breast, sliced into thin strips

2 fresh plum tomatoes, diced

¼ cup fresh dill, chopped

¼ cup fresh parsley, chopped

¼ cup fresh mint

In a saucepan, combine the broth, garlic, carrots, parsnips, celery, and onions.

Bring to a boil over high heat. Reduce to low and simmer for 6 minutes.

Turn the heat to high and add the lemon juice and noodles. Cook for 5 minutes. Add the chicken and cook for another 4 minutes.

Remove from the heat and add the plum tomatoes, dill, parsley, and mint. Serve hot.

MAKES 6 SERVINGS

NUTRITIONAL VALUES PER SERVING: calories—211, fat—5 grams, protein—19 grams, carbohydrates—19 grams

Potato Casserole

2 pounds potatoes, peeled and
   diced
6 plum tomatoes, diced
2 small onions, diced

3 cloves garlic, minced
3 teaspoons thyme
2 cups low-sodium chicken broth

Preheat the oven to 375 degrees.

In a large bowl, mix the potatoes, tomatoes, onions, garlic, thyme, and salt and pepper to taste.

Place in a shallow casserole pan.

Pour the broth over the vegetables and bake uncovered for approximately 1 hour, or until the potatoes are tender and the broth is absorbed.

MAKES 8 SERVINGS

NUTRITIONAL VALUES PER SERVING: calories—157, protein—4.3 grams, fat—less than 1 gram, carbohydrates—29.6 grams

Twice-Baked Potatoes with Broccoli and/or Carrots

6 potatoes
2 cups diced carrots or 2 cups
   broccoli, chopped (or both)
3 tablespoons Dijon mustard

¼ cup chopped fresh dill
½ cup low-fat yogurt
¼ cup 1% milk
¼ cup Parmesan cheese

Preheat the oven to 400 degrees. Prick each potato several times.

Bake the potatoes for 1 hour, or until soft. Meanwhile, steam the carrots and/or broccoli until soft, about 10 minutes. In a food processor, puree the carrots and/or broccoli with mustard, ¼ cup dill, and ¼ cup yogurt. Set the vegetable puree aside. Cut each cooked potato in half lengthwise. Scoop the potatoes out of the skins and put in a bowl. Mash with milk, then add the pureed mixture and stir. Put the entire mixture back into the skins and sprinkle with Parmesan cheese. Lower the oven temperature to 350 degrees and bake for approximately 20 minutes, or until the tops are browned.

MAKES 6 SERVINGS
NUTRITIONAL VALUES PER SERVING: calories—170, protein—6.5 grams, fat—2 grams, carbohydrates—32 grams

Low-fat Risotto

2 cloves garlic, minced
1 small onion or 4–5 shallots,
    chopped
1 tablespoon olive oil
6 cups low-sodium chicken broth

1½ cups Arborio rice
Salt and pepper
Parmesan cheese, thyme, rosemary,
    or steamed vegetables (optional)

In a heavy saucepan, sauté the garlic and onion in olive oil until soft, 5 minutes. In another saucepan, heat the broth until simmering. Add the rice to the garlic and onion mixture and stir for 2 minutes. Add ¼ cup broth to the rice and stir on low heat until the broth is absorbed. Repeat this process, adding ¼ cup broth at a time, until all the broth is used. Total cooking time is approximately 30 minutes (keep stirring).

Add salt and pepper to taste.

Serve alone or sprinkle with 1 tablespoon Parmesan cheese and/or herbs such as thyme or rosemary.

You can also top with steamed vegetables such as mushrooms, peppers, zucchini, asparagus, or squash. Add the vegetables to the last 2 cups of broth and steam. Add to the rice.

MAKES 6 SERVINGS
NUTRITIONAL VALUES PER SERVING: calories—137, fat—4 grams (if tablespoon Parmesan cheese is added, add 1.5 grams of fat), protein—7 grams, carbohydrates—18 grams

THE BLENDER: A NEW MOM'S BEST FRIEND

Forget diamonds. A blender can be your new best friend. Sometimes you are hungry and you know that you need to eat something nutritious, but you are just too tired or too busy to prepare a regular meal for yourself. The solution? How about three awesome "health shakes" that are as easy to make as they are tasty? Each shake packs tremendous nutritional wallop and can be used to replace an occasional meal if need be. The first step is to go to a health food store and purchase a can of either soy protein powder or *spirulina*, a vegetable-based protein powder. They come in different flavors, but I recommend that you buy the vanilla flavor, because it blends best with other ingredients. There are different grades of protein powders, depending on their protein content. You should buy the high-grade variety that contains over 90 percent protein. Get out your blender and have some fun!

Banana Rama

3 heaping tablespoons protein powder

1 cup of skim milk

½ cup pineapple or orange juice

1 ripe banana

Blend all the ingredients for 1 minute.

MAKES 2 LARGE PORTIONS. SERVE WITH ICE.
NUTRITIONAL VALUES PER SERVING: total calories—180, calories from carbohydrates—100, calories from protein—70, calories from fat—10

Chocolate Fudge Attack

2 heaping tablespoons protein powder

½ cup Edy's low-fat chocolate fudge ice cream

½ cup skim milk

2 cups ice cubes

Blend all the ingredients for 1 minute

MAKES 1 PORTION
NUTRITIONAL VALUES PER SERVING: total calories—225, calories from carbohydrates—100, calories from protein—95, calories from fat—30

Orange Cream

8 ounces orange juice
1 cup Dannon nonfat vanilla yogurt
2 heaping tablespoons protein
   powder

2 cups ice cubes
½ cup water

Blend all the ingredients in a blender for 45 seconds.

MAKES 1 SERVING

NUTRITIONAL VALUES PER SERVING: total calories—270, calories from carbohydrates—150, calories from protein—100, calories from fat—20

Part V

Eating in
the Fast Lane

Chapter Eleven

Eating in the Fast Lane: A New Mom's Survival Guide

"Billions and billions and billions served." I know that I didn't eat all those hamburgers, so it must be you! If billions of hamburgers have been eaten, then billions of French fries also must have sailed over the counter and into our bellies. Fast food has become a fixture not only in America but around the world. One only has to travel to Europe, the Far East, and even the Middle East, to see how American fast food has replaced the automobile as *the* American export. What is the first thing that visitors from countries with world-class cuisine like France and Italy want to do when they step off the plane? Go to a fast-food restaurant, of course!

Fast food, as a product, is all about taste, and the taste of the food comes from fat. Take out the "s" from the word "fast" and you are left with *fat*. Fat gets loaded into everything served, from burgers and fries to vegetables, chicken, and even fish, as you shall see.

In Japan, where fast food is relatively new, scientists have measured the cholesterol levels of people who live near and far away from a fast-food restaurant. Those who live closest have the highest cholesterol levels. Those who live furthest away have the lowest cholesterol levels. Japan has always had a lower incidence of cholesterol-related heart problems and obesity than we do. But guess what? Since the introduction of fast food, the incidence of obesity and heart disease is climbing in Japan!

I know that sooner or later there is a good chance you will find yourself in a fast-food emporium. During the first trimester of pregnancy, you might stop in to satiate your craving for high-fat, salty, juicy, high-calorie foods. Later, in the third trimester and after delivery, fast food can help you avoid standing on your achy legs cooking the family a six-course dinner. Who has time for that? Fast food is even easier than home-delivered food for a new mom because there is no table to set, nor dishes to wash.

There is nothing wrong with eating fast food once or twice a week, but no more than that. Moreover, *Hello, Baby! Good-bye Baby Fat!* believes that when you go fast-food, what you put into your mouth should blend with the postpartum weight loss plan we have discussed. You already know that portion control is the key to long-term weight loss success. If there is any place in the world where portions take a holiday, it's in fast-food restaurants. I have two rules regarding portion control in fast-food restaurants. First, if you need two hands to hold it and two hands to eat it, it's not right for you. Second, stay away from any hamburger or sandwich that has its own name!

If you find that controlling portion size is too hard, you can make up for it by watching how much fat you ingest.

There are a myriad of fast-food choices. Some choices are deceptively fat-laden, while other choices are healthier. For instance, if I were to ask you which is a healthier choice in terms of fat content and calories—a large Taco Salad with Ranch Dressing (Taco Bell) or a Big Mac (McDonald's)—you probably would say the salad would be the healthier choice. After all, how can you "kill" a healthy salad? It's apparently a lot easier than you think. Just add a nice fatty dressing like ranch dressing. That Taco Salad with Ranch Dressing contains 1000 calories and 87 grams of fat, of which 45 percent is saturated fat, the bad stuff for your heart. The Big Mac, on the other hand, is a far healthier choice at 500 calories and "only" 26 grams of fat. It's all relative!

To help you navigate your way through the fast-food minefield, we have prepared a sampling of menus from the more popular restaurants. Next to each food choice, we list the amount of total calories and fat calories for each food. It would serve you well to try and adhere to the 30 percent fat rule when selecting among fast foods, and it can be done. You should try and limit your daily fat intake to 500 calories (about 55 grams of fat), or, if you are nursing, you should limit your daily fat intake to about 650 calories from fat (about 70 grams of fat). Some single fast-food entrées come close to and actually exceed these numbers by themselves! Learn which ones you should stay away from.

Let's begin with two special lists that we have prepared for you: the "best of" and the "worst of" popular national fast-food chains. The criteria for inclusion in the "worst of" category is simply to be a high-fat version of a food that you think should be healthy and relatively low-fat. Therefore, the "worst of" list contains salads, vegetables, fish, and chicken dishes. You are going to be surprised! I know I was. Did you know that one packet of Newman's Own ranch dressing served at Burger King contains 350 calories and 37 grams of fat and is, in fact, 95 percent fat? The only food substances that contain more fat than that are lard and butter! The "best of" list contains some surprises as well, but this time the surprises are in your favor. You'll find some very tasty choices that you think would be high in fat but aren't. These are the types of foods that we encourage you to select when you eat fast foods.

There are few breakfast or dessert offerings on our list, and the reason is simple. Finding a healthy breakfast or dessert choice in a fast-food restaurant is indeed the ultimate oxymoron. Only an "ox" of inferior intelligence would look for one there, anyway!

Check out our fast-food lists before you venture to the food court at the mall so that you can make smart choices for yourself—like staying home and having your husband or boyfriend cook for you!

Fast-Food Charts

The "Worst of" Fast Foods

The "Best of" Fast Foods

Calorie Counts
for Fast-Food Restaurant Menus

THE "WORST OF" FAST FOOD . . .

The Salad Myth (Did You Say Salad?)

- *Taco Salad with Ranch Dressing (Taco Bell)*: 1167 calories, 783 fat calories (67% fat calories)
- *Seafood Salad with Ranch Dressing (Taco Bell)*: 884 calories, 594 fat calories (67% fat calories)
- *Caesar Salad with Chicken (Boston Market)*: 670 calories, 423 fat calories (63% fat calories)
- *Caesar Salad Entree (Boston Market)*: 520 calories, 387 fat calories (58% fat calories)
- *Newman's Own Ranch Dressing (Burger King)*, 1 packet: 350 calories, 333 fat calories (95% fat calories)

Sounds Fishy . . .

- *Fish Sandwich (Wendy's)*: 460 calories, 225 fat calories (49% fat calories)
- *Fillet-O-Fish (McDonald's)*: 370 calories, 162 fat calories (44% fat calories)
- *Tuna Melt (Little Caesars)*: 700 calories, 333 fat calories (48% fat calories)

Eat Your Vegetables . . . But Not These

- *Vegetarian Sandwich (Little Caesars)*: 620 calories, 270 fat calories (44% fat calories)
- *Veggie Pizza with Salad (Little Caesars)*: 640 calories, 198 fat calories (31% fat calories)
- *Veggie and Cheese Italian Sub (Subway)*: 535 calories, 153 fat calories (29% fat calories)
- *Onion Rings (Burger King)*: 339 calories, 171 fat calories (50% fat calories)
- *Baked Potato with Sour Cream and Chives (Wendy's)*: 500 calories, 207 fat calories (41% fat calories)
- *Croissant Sandwich with Mushrooms and Cheese (Arby's)*: 493 calories, 342 fat calories (69% fat calories)

Chicken . . . Cluck, Cluck on This

- *Chicken Sandwich (Burger King)*: 685 calories, 360 fat calories (53% fat calories)
- *Chunky Chicken Salad Sandwich (Boston Market)*: 640 calories, 279 fat calories (44% fat calories)
- *Chicken Pot Pie (Boston Market)*: 750 calories, 306 fat calories (41% fat calories)
- *Chicken Nuggets, 6 (McDonald's)*: 270 calories, 135 fat calories (50% fat calories)
- *Chicken Thigh, Extra Crispy (KFC)*: 370 calories, 225 fat calories (61% fat calories)
- *Hot Chicken Wings, 6 (KFC)*: 471 calories, 297 fat calories (63% fat calories)

Fast Food Is Not for Breakfast Anymore

- *Biscuit, Plain (Burger King)*: 332 calories, 153 fat calories (46% fat calories)
- *Bagel with Sausage, Egg, and Cheese (Burger King)*: 626 calories, 324 fat calories (52% fat calories)
- *French Toastix, 3.5 ounces (Arby's)*: 420 calories, 225 fat calories (54% fat calories)
- *Crescent (Roy Rogers)*: 408 calories, 243 fat calories (60% fat calories)

Did You Say "Side Dish" or "Main Dish"?

- *Cranberry Relish, ¾ cup (Boston Market)*: 370 calories, 45 fat calories (12% fat calories)
- *Creamed Spinach, ¾ cup (Boston Market)*: 300 calories, 144 fat calories (48% fat calories)
- *Corn on the Cob, 5.3 ounces (KFC)*: 222 calories, 108 fat calories (49% fat calories)
- *Corn Bread, 2 ounces (KFC)*: 228 calories, 117 fat calories (51% fat calories)
- *Macaroni Salad, 3.8 ounces (KFC)*: 248 calories, 153 fat calories (62% fat calories)

• *Tortellini Salad,* ¾ cup (*Boston Market*): 380 calories, 216 fat calories (57% fat calories)

It Is What It Is . . .

• *French Fries,* large order (*McDonald's*): 320 calories, 153 fat calories (48% fat calories)
• *Cold-Cut Sub,* foot-long (*Subway*): 853 calories, 360 fat calories (42% fat calories)
• *Whopper* (*Burger King*): 614 calories, 324 fat calories (53% fat calories)
• *Big Mac* (*McDonald's*): 500 calories, 234 fat calories (47% fat calories)

THE "BEST OF" FAST FOOD

Olé!

• *Light Taco Salad without Chips* (*Taco Bell*): 330 calories, 81 fat calories (25% fat calories)
• *Light Taco* (*Taco Bell*): 140 calories, 45 fat calories (32% fat calories)
• *Light Bean Burrito* (*Taco Bell*): 330 calories, 54 fat calories (16% fat calories)
• *Chicken Fajita* (*Taco Bell*): 226 calories, 90 fat calories (40% fat calories)
• *Chili,* 9 ounces (*Wendy's*): 220 calories, 63 fat calories (29% fat calories)

Chick, Chick, Hooray!

• ¼ *Chicken, White, without Skin* (*Boston Market*): 160 calories, 36 fat calories (23% fat calories)
• *Chicken Breast and Wing without Skin* (*Roy Rogers*): 190 calories, 54 fat calories (28% fat calories)
• *Grilled Chicken Deluxe* (*McDonald's*): 330 calories, 54 fat calories (16% fat calories)

- *Chunky Chicken Salad (Burger King)*: 142 calories, 36 fat calories (25% fat calories)
- *Roast Chicken Salad (Arby's)*: 204 calories, 65 fat calories (32% fat calories)
- *Chicken Breast Sandwich (Boston Market)*: 420 calories, 45 fat calories (11% fat calories)
- *BBQ Chicken Sandwich (KFC)*: 256 calories, 72 fat calories (28% fat calories)
- *Grilled Chicken Salad (Wendy's)*: 200 calories, 72 fat calories (36% fat calories)
- *Chicken Soup (Boston Market)*: 80 calories, 27 fat calories (34% fat calories)
- *Chicken Noodle Soup (Arby's)*: 99 calories, 16 fat calories (16% fat calories)

Sides That Won't Stick to Your Sides

- *Rice Pilaf, ⅔ cup (Boston Market)*: 180 calories, 45 fat calories (25% fat calories)
- *New Potatoes, ¾ cup (Boston Market)*: 140 calories, 27 fat calories (19% fat calories)
- *Red Beans and Rice, 3.9 ounces (KFC)*: 114 calories, 27 fat calories (24% fat calories)
- *Mashed Potatoes (KFC)*: 59 calories, 0 fat
- *Crazy Bread (Little Caesars)*: 98 calories, 9 fat calories (9% fat calories)
- *Garden Salad (McDonald's)*: 50 calories, 18 fat calories (36% fat calories)
- *Salad Dressing, Vinaigrette (McDonald's)*: 12 calories, 4.5 fat calories (38% fat calories)
- *Baked Potato (Wendy's)*: 270 calories, 0 fat

Sandwiches and Such

- *Turkey Sandwich, Plain (Boston Market)*: 440 calories, 72 fat calories (16% fat calories)
- *Turkey Sandwich, Light Roast Deluxe (Arby's)*: 294 calories, 54 fat calories (18% fat calories)

- *Turkey Sandwich*, 6-inch (*Subway*): 357 calories, 90 fat calories (25% fat calories)
- *Regular Hamburger* (*McDonald's*): 255 calories, 81 fat calories (32% fat calories)
- *Light Roast Beef Sandwich* (*Arby's*): 294 calories, 90 fat calories (31% fat calories)
- *Roast Beef Sandwich* (*Roy Rogers*): 350 calories, 99 fat calories (28% fat calories)
- *Veggie Pot Pie* (*Boston Market*): 350 calories, 108 fat calories (31% fat calories)
- *Cheese Pizza Slice*, 2.2 ounces (*Little Caesars*): 170 calories, 54 fat calories (32% fat calories)

CALORIE COUNTS FOR FAST-FOOD RESTAURANT MENUS

McDONALD'S

FOOD	CALORIES	FAT CALORIES
BISCUIT	260	117
BISCUIT W/SAUSAGE & EGG	505	297
QUARTER POUNDER	410	180
QUARTER POUNDER W/CHEESE	510	252
HAMBURGER	255	81
CHEESEBURGER	305	117
CHICKEN SANDWICH	415	171
GRILLED CHICKEN DELUXE	330	54
CHICKEN NUGGETS, 6 PIECES	270	135
FISH SANDWICH	370	162
BIG MAC	500	234
FRENCH FRIES, LARGE	320	153
CHEF'S SALAD, 9.5 OUNCES	170	81
CHUNKY CHICKEN SALAD, 9 OUNCES	150	36
GARDEN SALAD, 6.7 OUNCES	50	36
VINAIGRETTE	12	4.5
THOUSAND ISLAND DRESSING	78	72
MILLKSHAKE, CHOCOLATE	320	15

BURGER KING

FOOD	CALORIES	FAT CALORIES
BAGEL W/SAUSAGE, EGG & CHEESE	626	324
HAMBURGER	272	99
CHEESEBURGER	318	135
WHOPPER	614	324
WHOPPER W/CHEESE	706	396
DOUBLE WHOPPER W/CHEESE	935	549
WHOPPER JR.	330	171
WHOPPER JR. W/CHEESE	380	198
CHICKEN SANDWICH	685	360
CHICKEN BROILER	379	162
CHICKEN TENDERS, 6 PIECES	236	117
FISH SANDWICH	495	225
FRENCH FRIES, MEDIUM	372	180
ONION RINGS	339	171
CHEF'S SALAD	178	81
CHUNKY CHICKEN SALAD	142	36
GARDEN SALAD	95	45
'NEWMAN'S OWN' REDUCED CALORIE ITALIAN DRESSING, 1 PKT.	170	162
'NEWMAN'S OWN' RANCH DRESSING, 1 PKT.	350	333

BOSTON MARKET

FOOD	CALORIES	FAT CALORIES
CAESAR SALAD W/CHICKEN	670	423
CAESAR SALAD ENTREE	520	387
CHICKEN BREAST SANDWICH	420	45
CHUNKY CHICKEN SALAD SANDWICH	640	279
CHICKEN SOUP	80	27
¼ DARK MEAT CHICKEN W/SKIN	330	198
¼ DARK MEAT CHICKEN W/O SKIN	210	90
¼ WHITE MEAT CHICKEN W/SKIN	330	153
¼ WHITE MEAT CHICKEN W/O SKIN	160	36
CHICKEN POT PIE	750	306
VEGETABLE POT PIE	350	108
TURKEY SANDWICH, PLAIN	440	72
CRANBERRY RELISH, ¾ CUP	370	45
BAKED BEANS, ¾ CUP	330	81
CREAMED SPINACH, ¾ CUP	300	216
NEW POTATOES, ¾ CUP	140	27
MASHED POTATOES, ⅔ CUP	180	72
RICE PILAF, ⅔ CUP	180	45
STUFFING, ¾ CUP	310	108
CORN BREAD, 2.4 OUNCES	200	54
COLESLAW, ¾ CUP	280	144
TORTELLINI SALAD, ¾ CUP	380	216
MEDITERRANEAN SALAD, ¾ CUP	170	90

WENDY'S

FOOD	CALORIES	FAT CALORIES
BREAKAST SANDWICH	370	171
BIG CLASSIC BURGER ON KAISER BUN	470	225
SINGLE BURGER ON BUN, ¼ POUND	350	144
SINGLE BURGER W/EVERYTHING	420	189
DOUBLE CHEESEBURGER	620	324
CHEESEBURGER JR.	310	117
CHICKEN SANDWICH, GRILLED	340	117
CHICKEN SANDWICH, FRIED	440	171
CHICKEN NUGGETS, 6 PIECES	310	189
FISH SANDWICH	460	225
STEAK SANDWICH	440	225
BAKED POTATO, PLAIN	270	0
BAKED POTATO W/BROCCOLI & CHEESE	400	144
BAKED POTATO W/SOUR CREAM/CHIVE	500	207
CHILI, 9 OUNCES	220	63
FRENCH FRIES, REGULAR	300	135
CAESAR SALAD, SIDE	160	54
CHEF'S SALAD, 9.1 OUNCES	130	45
GRILLED CHICKEN SALAD	200	72

LITTLE CAESARS

FOOD	CALORIES	FAT CALORIES
CHEESE PIZZA, SLICE	170	54
CHEESE PIZZA ENTREE W/SALAD	600	189
VEGGIE PIZZA ENTREE W/SALAD	640	198
BABY PAN PIZZA	525	198
CRAZY BREAD	98	9
ANTIPASTO SALAD W/LO-CAL DRESSING	170	81
GREEK SALAD W/LO-CAL DRESSING	140	72
ITALIAN SUB	590	252
TUNA MELT	700	333
TURKEY SANDWICH	450	153
VEGETARIAN SANDWICH	620	270

KENTUCKY FRIED CHICKEN (KFC)

FOOD	CALORIES	FAT CALORIES
CHICKEN BREAST, 'EXTRA TASTY CRISPY'	342	180
CHICKEN BREAST, 'ORIG. RECIPE'	260	126
CHICKEN BREAST, 'SKIN-FREE CRISPY'	296	144
DRUMSTICK, 'EXTRA TASTY CRISPY'	190	99
DRUMSTICK, 'ORIG. RECIPE'	130	63
DRUMSTICK, 'SKIN-FREE CRISPY'	166	81
THIGH, 'EXTRA TASTY CRISPY'	370	225
THIGH, 'ORIG. RECIPE'	260	153
THIGH, 'SKIN-FREE CRISPY'	256	153
WING, 'EXTRA TASTY CRISPY'	200	117
WING, 'ORIG. RECIPE'	150	72
HOT WINGS, 6 PIECES	471	297
CHICKEN NUGGETS, 6 PIECES	284	162
COLONEL'S CHICKEN SAND., 5.9 OUNCES	482	243
BBQ CHICKEN SAND., 5.3 OUNCES	256	72
FRENCH FRIES, REG., 2.7 OUNCES	244	108
POTATO WEDGES, 3.3 OUNCES	192	81
MASHED POTATOES	59	0
RED BEANS AND RICE, 3.9 OUNCES	114	27
MACARONI & CHEESE, 4 OUNCES	162	72
CORN ON THE COB, 5.3 OUNCES	222	108
CORN BREAD, 2 OUNCES	228	117
MACARONI SALAD, 3.8 OUNCES	248	153
POTATO SALAD, 4.4 OUNCES	180	99
GARDEN SALAD, 3.1 OUNCES	16	0
ITALIAN SALAD DRESSING, 1 OUNCE	15	9
RANCH SALAD DRESSING, 1 OUNCE	170	162

SUBWAY

FOOD	CALORIES	FAT CALORIES
COLD CUT SUB, ITALIAN ROLL, FT LONG	853	360
HAM, 6 INCH	360	99
HAM & CHEESE, ITALIAN, FT LONG	643	162
ITALIAN MEATBALL, FT LONG	917	396
ROAST BEEF, 6 INCH	375	99
ROAST BEEF, ITALIAN, FT LONG	689	207
SEAFOOD AND CRAB, 6 INCH	388	108
STEAK & CHEESE, ITALIAN, FT LONG	765	288
TUNA, 6 INCH	402	117
TURKEY, 6 INCH	357	90
TURKEY, ITALIAN, FT LONG	645	171
VEGGIES & CHEESE, ITALIAN, FT LONG	535	153
CHEF'S SALAD, SMALL	189	90
GARDEN SALAD, LARGE	46	0
SALAD DRESSING, LITE ITALIAN, 4 TABLESPOONS	23	0

TACO BELL

FOOD	CALORIES	FAT CALORIES
BELLGRANDE NACHOS, 10.1 OUNCES	649	315
SUPREME NACHOS, 5.1 OUNCES	367	243
REGULAR NACHOS, 3.7 OUNCES	346	162
SEAFOOD SALAD W/RANCH DRESSING	884	594
SEAFOOD SALAD W/O DRESSING	648	378
SEAFOOD SALAD W/O DRESSING, W/O SHELL	217	99
TACO SALAD, 21 OUNCES	905	549
TACO SALAD W/RANCH DRESSING	1167	783
TACO SALAD W/O BEANS	822	513
TACO SALAD W/O SHELL	484	279
LIGHT TACO SALAD W/CHIPS, 19.11 OUNCES	680	225
LIGHT TACO SALAD W/O CHIPS, 16.57 OUNCES	330	81
SALAD DRESSING, RANCH, 2.6 OUNCES	236	225
SALSA, 0.34 OUNCE	18	0
SOUR CREAM, 0.75 OUNCE	46	36
BELLGRANDE TACO, 5.7 OUNCES	335	207
CHICKEN TACO, 3 OUNCES	171	81
LIGHT TACO, 2.79 OUNCES	140	45
PLATTER, LIGHT	1062	522
REGULAR TACO, 2.75 OUNCES	183	99
SUPREME TACO, 3.25 OUNCES	230	135
MEXICAN PIZZA, 7.9 OUNCES	575	333
BEEF TOSTADA	322	180

TACO BELL

CHICKEN TOSTADA W/RED SAUCE, 5.8 OUNCES	264	135
CHICKEN TOSTADA W/RED SAUCE, 5.5 OUNCES	243	99
CHICKEN FAJITA	226	90
BEAN BURRITO, 7.3 OUNCES	447	126
BEEF BURRITO, 7.3 OUNCES	493	189
CHICKEN BURRITO, 6 OUNCES	334	108
SUPREME BURRITO, 9 OUNCES	503	198
LIGHT BEAN BURRITO, 7.07 OUNCES	330	54
LIGHT SUPREME BURRITO, 8.86 OUNCES	503	198
LIGHT 7-LAYER BURRITO, 9.53 OUNCES	440	81

ROY ROGERS

FOOD	CALORIES	FAT CALORIES
BISCUIT	231	108
EGG & BISCUIT PLATTER	557	306
EGG & BISCUIT PLATTER W/SAUSAGE	713	441
CRESCENT	408	243
CHICKEN BREAST, FRIED	412	216
CHICKEN BREAST & WING W/O SKIN	190	54
CHICKEN LEG, FRIED	140	72
CHICKEN LEG & THIGH, FRIED	436	252
CHICKEN NUGGETS, FRIED, 6 PIECES	288	162
FISH SANDWICH	514	216
FRENCH FRIES, REGULAR	320	144
HAMBURGER, EXPRESS	561	288
HAMBURGER, REGULAR	472	225
HAMBURGER, ROY ROGERS BAR	573	279
HAMBURGER, SMALL	222	81
CHEESEBURGER, EXPRESS	613	333
CHEESEBURGER, REGULAR	525	261
CHEESEBURGER, SMALL	275	117
CHEESEBURGER W/BACON	552	297
ROAST BEEF SANDWICH, LARGE	373	108
ROAST BEEF SANDWICH, LARGE W/CHEESE	427	153
ROAST BEEF SANDWICH, REGULAR	350	99
ROAST BEEF SANDWICH, REG W/CHEESE	403	135
GREEK PASTA SALAD, ¼ CUP	159	81
MACARONI SALAD, ¼ CUP	93	45
POTATO SALAD, ¼ CUP	54	27
BAKED POTATO, PLAIN	211	0

ARBY'S

FOOD	CALORIES	FAT CALORIES
FRENCH TOASTIX, 3.5 OUNCES	420	225
CROISSANT SANDWICH, W/MUSHROOM & CHEESE	493	342
ARBY Q SANDWICH	389	135
FRENCH DIP SANDWICH	526	243
ROAST BEEF SANDWICH, LIGHT DELUXE	294	90
ROAST BEEF SANDWICH, REGULAR	383	171
ROAST BEEF SANDWICH, SUPER	552	261
ITALIAN SUB	671	351
TUNA SUB	663	333
TURKEY SUB	486	171
TURKEY SANDWICH, LIGHT ROAST DELUXE	260	54
FISH SANDWICH	526	243
CHICKEN SANDWICH, FILLET	445	207
CHICKEN SANDWICH, GRILLED, BBQ	386	117
FRENCH FRIES, CHEDDAR	399	198
FRENCH FRIES, CURLY	337	162
DELUXE BAKED POTATO	621	324
POTATO SOUP, W/BACON	184	81
CHICKEN NOODLE SOUP	99	18
CHEESE SOUP	281	162
SALAD, ROAST CHICKEN	204	63
SALAD, CHEF'S	205	85
SALAD DRESSING, LIGHT ITALIAN	23	10
SALAD DRESSING, BUTTERMILK RANCH	349	347

The Future of Weight Loss

New moms get to watch lots of old movies. For one reason or another, you will find yourself awake at some ungodly hour, watching T.V., and old movies rule the airwaves at night. Movies often end with people saying good-bye to each other, and many movies have the word good-bye in the title. There's *The Long Goodbye; The Goodbye People; Goodbye, Mr. Chips; Goodbye Charlie; Goodbye, My Fancy; Goodbye Norma Jean; Good-bye, My Lady; Goodbye, Columbus; Goodbye, New York; Kiss Me Goodbye;* and my favorite: *The Goodbye Girl*. That reminds me: It is time for us to say good-bye.

The months have passed quickly. Now a veteran mom, I'm sure you are eager to pass your child-rearing wisdom and experience on to the next generation. Your child, who weighed just a few pounds several months ago, is now racing past every physical milestone on the pediatrician's chart. Mom, you too have reached a milestone. Your body has changed forever, both inside and out. Consider this: More than likely, the *least* you will weigh as an adult is what you weigh right now, and you want to hold on to your success.

Even though your special postpartum weight loss advantage has ended, a brand-new phase has begun that will last for the rest of your life. To keep weight off, you need to maintain constant vigilance. Each and every day, you should be doing the things that brought you weight loss success in the first place. Whether you are a thin Type A new mom or the heaviest Type C new mom, one thing is certain: the lessons learned from your three trimesters of weight loss can cement your weight loss success in the future. In fact, no matter what you weigh, one important weight loss lesson can be gleaned from each trimester of weight loss that will keep you thinner in the years ahead.

From the first trimester of weight loss, you learned that cutting back on your fat intake is a key to losing weight. Keeping your fat intake down from now on is just as important. A new study from the University of Auckland, New Zealand, found that the people who were most likely to sustain weight loss were those who made the largest reductions in their fat intake! We still have a long way to go before the optimal weight loss diet is established, assuming that one even exists. In the meantime, it's back to common sense and a scale one more time. Avoid all fad diets. No diet is better than *yours*, because yours is the one that keeps you alive and happy. Your job now is to continue what you have already been doing over the past few months. That is, modify your diet by doing two things at every meal: (1) control portion sizes, and (2) limit fat to 30 percent total fat calories per day.

Never deprive yourself or starve yourself. (A woman once told me that she was on *five* diets. "Why five diets?" I asked her. "I don't get enough food from one diet!" she replied.)

Don't wait for the next miracle weight loss diet. Your new understanding about yourself should tell you that the only true miracle is how amazing your body is!

From the second trimester of weight loss, you know that in order to be in sync with your body, you must learn to go to sleep on an empty stomach. I can't tell you how many women right now are totally out of control, munching on fatty foods late at night that linger in their stomachs until morning. (Not you, because you know better.) This is one key to weight loss success that, with a little practice, becomes easier over time.

From the third trimester of weight loss comes your third cornerstone of lifelong weight control: exercise. As you already know, it plays no role in postpartum weight loss (unless you are an obese new mom who nurses), but exercise will play a large role in keeping your future weight down. A multitude of studies have all reached a similar conclusion: To maintain lifelong weight loss success, some form of habitual physical movement is required.

One of the great joys of motherhood is watching your child's motor skills progress. From relatively inert bundles that need to be carried, they are soon holding their heads high. Next they roll, sit up, crawl, and walk with assistance. Then one day your child is walking by himself or herself—the first sure sign of physical independence. Running soon follows. From the look of joy on your baby's face, it is obvious that life is not complete without movement. Life *is* movement!

Recapture the same smile that once spread across your face when you were the child who began to walk. Put more movement into your life by finding a physical activity that you enjoy. It need not involve a glider, rider, strider, or roller. Keep it simple, like walking, gardening, stretching, dancing, or doing yoga. You don't have to sweat or worry about getting your heart rate up to some targeted level. Your commitment to daily exercise of any kind, at any intensity, is far more important. Challenge yourself. Experiment. Try things that you've never done before. Get into a daily rhythm that involves sustained movement. Whatever activities you choose, use them as a foundation on which you plan and establish your own personal time-out. Don't wait for a break in your busy schedule. Make your own break! Fifteen to twenty minutes' worth of exercise each day is all it takes to reenergize your spiritual and physical batteries.

Keep moving, Mom. To keep that fresh, young, new-mom spirit inside you alive always, you don't have to be a baby; just act like one!

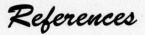

References

Part I: New Baby, New Body

Boardley, D., et al. Postpartum weight change: The relationship between diet, activity and other factors, and postpartum weight change by race. *Obstetrics and Gynecology* (1995) 86 (5): 834–38.

Caulfield, L., et al. Race and maternal weight gain: Determinants of gestational weight gain outside the recommended ranges among black and white women. *Obstetrics and Gynecology* (1996) 87 (5 Pt 1): 760–766.

Dennis, K. J., et al. Changes in body weight after delivery. *Journal of Obstetrics and Gynecology* (1965) 72: 94–102.

Dugdale, A., Eaton-Evans, J. The effect of lactation and other factors on postpartum changes in body weight and triceps skin-fold thickness. *British Journal of Nutrition* (1989) 61: 149–153.

Greene, G., et al. Post-partum weight change: How much of the weight gained in pregnancy will be lost after delivery? *Obstetrics and Gynecology* (1988) 71 (5): 701–707.

Huang, Z., et al. Body weight, weight change, and risk for hypertension in women. *Annals of Internal Medicine* (1998) 128: 81–88.

Kassirer, J., Angell, M. Losing weight: An ill-fated New Year's resolution. *New England Journal of Medicine* (1998) 338: 52–54.

Kawakami, S., et al. Alteration of maternal body weight in pregnancy and postpartum. *Keio Journal of Medicine* (1977) 26 (62): 53–62.

Lederman, S. A. Reproduction and obesity: The effect of pregnancy weight gain on later obesity. *Obstetrics and Gynecology* (1993) 82 (1): 148–155.

McKeown, T., Record, R. The influence of reproduction on body weight in women. *Journal of Endocrinology* (1957) 15: 393–409.

Ohlin, A., Rosser, S. Maternal body weight development after pregnancy. *International Journal of Obesity* (1990) 14: 159–173.

Parker, J., Abrams, B. Postpartum weight retention: Differences in postpartum weight retention between black and white mothers. *Obstetrics and Gynecology* (1993) 81 (5) 1: 768–773.

Rookus, M., et al. The effect of pregnancy on the body mass index 9 months postpartum in 49 women. *International Journal of Obesity* (1987) 11: 609–618.

Schauberger, C. W., et al. Factors that influence weight loss in the puerperium. *Obstetrics and Gynecology* (1992) 79: 424–429.

Scholl, T., et al. Gestation weight gain: Pregnancy outcome and postpartum weight retention. *Obstetrics and Gynecology* (1995) 86: 423–427.

Sherwin, B. Hormones, mood and cognitive functioning in post-menopausal women. Estrogen and mood. *Obstetrics and Gynecology* (1996) 87 (2): 20S–21S.

Smith, C., et al. Weight gain, parity and race: Longitudinal changes in adiposity associated with pregnancy. *Journal of the American Medical Association (JAMA)* (1994) 271: 1747–1751.

Stevens, J., et al. The effect of age on the association between body-mass index and mortality. *New England Journal of Medicine* (1998) 338: 1–7.

Part II: The Three Postpartum Trimesters of Weight Loss

Adair, L. S., Popkin, B. M. Prolonged lactation contributes to depletion of maternal energy reserves in Filipino women. *Journal of Nutrition* (1992) 122 (8): 1643–1655.

Ahema, R., et al. Leptin accelerates the onset of puberty in normal female mice. *Journal of Clinical Investigation* (1997) 99 (3): 391–395.

American Academy of Pediatrics, Work Group on Breastfeeding. Breastfeeding and the use of human milk (1997) *Pediatrics* 100 (6): 1035–1039.

Areias, M., et al. Comparative incidence of depression in women and men, during pregnancy and after childbirth. *British Journal of Psychiatry* (1996) 169: 30–35.

Areias, M., et al. Correlates of postnatal depression in mothers and fathers. *British Journal of Psychiatry* (1996) 169: 36–41.

Barash, I., et al. Leptin is a metabolic signal to the reproductive system. *Endocrinology* (1996) 137 (7): 3144–3147.

Brewer, M. M., Bates, M. R., Vannoy, L. P. Postpartum changes in maternal weight and body fat deposits in lactating vs. nonlactating women. *American Journal of Clinical Nutrition* (1989) 49: 259–265.

Calcium Supplements. *Medical Letter* (1996) 38: 108–109.

Caro, J., et al. Perspectives in diabetes: Leptin: The tale of an obesity gene. *Diabetes* (1996) 45: 1455–1462.

Cizza, G., et al. Pediatric endocrinology: High dose transdermal estrogen, corticotropin-releasing hormone, and post-natal depression. *Journal of Clinical Endocrinology and Metabolism* (1997) 82 (5): 704.

Connor, W., Connor, S. The case for a low-fat, high-carbohydrate diet. *New England Journal of Medicine* (1997) 337 (8): 562–563.

Depression in women. *ACOG Technical Bulletin* (1993) 182: 1–7

Dewey, K. G., Heinig, M. J., Nommsen, L. A. Maternal weight-loss pattern during prolonged lactation. *American Journal of Clinical Nutrition* (1993) 58: 162–166.

Dewey, K., McCrory, M. Effects of dieting and physical activity on pregnancy and lactation. *American Journal of Clinical Nutrition* (1994) 50 (suppl): 454S–464S.

Dusdieker, L., Hemingway, D., Stumbo, P. Is milk production impaired by dieting during lactation? *American Journal of Clinical Nutrition* (1994) 59: 833–840.

Eidelman, A., et al. Postpartum cognitive deficits: Cognitive deficits in women after childbirth. *Obstetrics and Gynecology* (1993): 81 (5 Pt 1): 764–766.

Fink, G., et al. Estrogen control of central neurotransmission: Effect on mood, mental state and memory. *Cellular and Molecular Neurobiology* (1996) 16: 325–344.

Fossey, L., et al. Postpartum blues: A clinical syndrome and predictor of post-natal depression. *Journal of Psychosomatic Obstetrics and Gynecology* (1997) 18: 17–21.

Grinspoon, S., et al. Effects of fasting and glucose infusion on basal and overnight leptin concentrations in normal-weight women. *American Journal of Clinical Nutrition* (1997) 66: 1352–1356.

Hachey, D. Benefits and risks of modifying maternal fat intake in pregnancy and lactation. *American Journal of Clinical Nutrition* (1994) 59 (suppl): 454S–464S.

Haffner, S. M., Mykkanen, L., Stern, MP. Leptin concentrations in women in the San Antonio Heart Study: Effect of menopausal status and postmenopausal hormone replacement therapy. *American Journal of Epidemiology* (1997) 146 (7): 581–585.

Hardie, L., et al. Circulating leptin in women: A longitudinal study in the menstrual cycle and during pregnancy. *Clinical Endocrinology Oxford* (1997) 47 (1): 101–106.

Harris, B., et al. Maternity blues and major endocrine changes: Cardiff puerperal mood and hormone study II. *British Medical Journal* (1994) 308: 949–953.

Helland, I., et al. leptin levels in pregnant women and newborn infants: Gender differences and reduction during the neonatal period. *Pediatrics* (1998) 101 (3): 465–466.

Hickey, M., et al. Gender-dependent effects of exercise training on serum leptin levels in humans. *American Journal of Physiology* (1997) 272 (4): E562–E566.

Hilson, J., Rasmussen, K., Kjolhede, C. Maternal obesity and breast-feeding success in rural population of white women. *American Journal of Clinical Nutrition* (1997) 66: 1371–1378.

Hipwell, A; Kumar, R. Maternal psychopathology and prediction of outcome based on mother-infant interaction ratings. *British Journal of Psychiatry* (1996) 169: 655–661.

Hirsch, J., et al. Diet composition and energy balance in humans. *American Journal of Clinical Nutrition*, (1998) 67 (suppl): 551S–555S.

Horns, P., Ratcliffe, L. Pregnancy outcomes among active and sedentary primiparous women. *Journal of Obstetrics and Gynecology* (1996) 25 (1): 49–54.

Horwood, L. J., Fergusson, D. Breastfeeding and later cognitive and academic outcomes. *Pediatrics* (1998) 101: 1.

Janney, C., Zhang, D., Sowers, M. Lactation and weight retention. *American Journal of Clinical Nutrition* (1997), 66: 1116–1123.

Katan, M., et al. Beyond low-fat diets. *New England Journal of Medicine* (1997) 337 (8): 563–566.

King, J., et al. Energy metabolism during pregnancy: Influence of maternal energy status. *American Journal of Clinical Nutrition* (1994) 59 (suppl): 439S–445S.

Knutson, B., et al. Selective alteration of personality and social behavior by serotonergic intervention. *American Journal of Psychiatry* (1998) 155: 373–378.

Leathers, S. J., et al. Postpartum degressive symptomatology in new mothers and fathers: Parenting, work and support. *Journal of Nervous and Mental Disorders* (1997) 185: 129–139.

Licinio, J., et al. Human leptin levels are pulsatile and inversely related to pituitary-adrenal function. *Nature Medicine* (1997) 3 (5): 575–579.

Lonnqvist, F., Wennlung, A., Arner, P. Relationship between circulating leptin and peripheral fat distribution in obese subjects. *International Journal of Obesity Related Metabolic Dissorders* (1997) 21 (4): 255–260.

Lovelady, C. A., Nommsen-Rivers, L. A., et al. Effects of exercise on plasma lipids and metabolism of lactating women. *Medicine and Science in Sports and Exercise* (1995) 27 (1): 22–28.

Lukas, M., et al. Letters: Serum cholesterol concentration and postpartum depression. *British Medical Journal* (1996) 314: 143–144.

Madhavapeddi, R., Rao, B. S. Energy balance in lactating undernourished Indian women. *European Journal of Clinical Nutrition* (1992) 46 (5): 349–354.

Marchini, G., et al. Plasma leptin in infants: Relations to birth weight and weight loss. *Pediatrics* (1998) 101 (3): 429–432.

Motil, K., et al. Lean body mass of well-nourished women is preserved during lactation. *American Journal of Clinical Nutrition* (1998) 67: 292–300.

Murray, L., et al. The cognitive development of 5-year old children of postnatally depressed mothers. *Journal of Child Psychology-Psychiatry* (1996) 37: 927–935.

Nagy, T. R., et al. Effects of gender, ethnicity, body composition and fat distribution on serum leptin concentrations in children. *Journal of Clinical Endocrinology and Metabolism* (1997) 82 (7): 2148–2152.

Niskanen, L., et al. Serum leptin in relation to resting energy expenditure and fuel metabolism in obese subjects. *International Journal of Obesity Related Metabolic Related Disorders* (1997) 21 (4): 309–319.

Potter, S., et al. Does infant feeding method influence maternal postpartum weight loss? *Journal of the American Dietetic Association* (1991) 91: 441–446.

Ranneries, C., et al. Fat metabolism in formerly obese women. *American Journal of Physiology* (1998) 274: E155–E161.

Reynolds, J. L. Post-traumatic stress disorder after childbirth: The phenomenon of traumatic birth. *Canadian Medical Association Journal* (1997) 156: 831–835.

Rojkittikhun, T., Einarsson, S., et al. Relationship between lactation-associated body weight loss, levels of metabolic and reproductive hormones and weaning-to-oestrous interval in primiparous sows. *Zentralbl Veterinarmed [A]* (1992) 39 (6): 426–432.

Rowe, L., Temple, S., Hawthorne, G. Mothers' emotional needs and difficulties after childbirth. *Australian Family Physician* (1996) 25: S53–S58.

Saad, M., et al. Diurnal and ultradian rhythmicity of plasma leptin: Effects of gender and adiposity. *Journal of Clinical Endocrinology and Metabolism* (1998) 83 (2): 453–459.

Schmidt, P. J., et al. Differential behavioral effects of gonadal steroids in women with and in those without premenstrual syndrome. *New England Journal of Medicine* (1998) 338: 209–216.

Senaris R., et al. Synthesis of leptin in human placenta. *Endocrinology* (1997) 138 (10): 4501–4504.

Sharp, D., et al. The impact of postnatal depression on boys' intellectual development. *Journal of Child Psychology and Psychiatry* (1995) 36: 1315–1336.

Sheikh, G. Observations of maternal weight behavior during puerperium. *American Journal of Obstetrics and Gynecology* (1971) 2: 244–250.

Shimizu, H., et al. Estrogen increases in vivo leptin production in rats and human subjects. *Journal of Endocrinology* (1997) 154 (2): 285–292.

Sichel, D., et al. Prophylactic estrogen in recurrent postpartum affective disorder. *Biological Psychiatry* (1995) 38: 814–818.

Susman, J. Postpartum depressive disorders. *Journal of Family Practice* (1996) 43 (6): S17–S24.

Treadway, C. R., et al. A psychoendocrine study of pregnancy and puerperium. *American Journal of Psychiatry* (1969) 125: 86–91.

Wade, G., et al. Leptin facilitates and inhibits sexual behavior in female hamsters. *American Journal of Physiology* (1997) 272 (4): R1354–R1358.

Walker, L. Predictors of weight gain at 6 and 18 months after childbirth: A pilot study. *Journal of Obstetrics and Gynecological Neonatal Nursing* (1996) 25 (1): 39–48.

Walther, V. Postpartum depression: A review for perinatal social workers. *Social Work Health Care* (1997) 24: 99–111.

Warner, R., et al. Demographic and obstetric risk factors for postnatal psychiatric morbidity. *British Journal of Psychiatry* (1996) 168: 607–611.

Willett, W. Is dietary fat a major determinant of body fat? *American Journal of Clinical Nutrition* (1998) 67 (suppl): 556S–562S.

Wisner, K., Stowe, Z. Psychobiology of postpartum mood disorders. *Seminars in Reproduction and Endocrinology* (1997) 15: 77–89.

Wisner, K., et al. Anti-depressant treatment during breast feeding. *American Journal of Psychiatry* (1997) 154 (8): 1174–1175.

Wilson Blackburn, M., Howes Galloway, D. Energy expenditure and consumption of mature, pregnant and lactating women. *Journal of the American Dietetic Association* (1976) 69: 29–37.

Part III: The Pregnancy XL Files

Abrams, B. Weight gain and energy intake during pregnancy. *Clinical Obstetrics and Gynecology* (1994) 37 (3): 515–527.

Abrams, B., Carmichael, S., Selvin, S. Factors associated with the pattern of maternal weight gain during pregnancy. *Obstetrics and Gynecology* (1995) 86 (2): 170–176.

ACOG Technical Bulletin. Nutrition during pregnancy. *American College of Obstetricians-Gynecologists* (April 1993) 179: 1–8.

Caan, B., Horgen, D., et al. Benefits associated with WIC supplemental feeding during the interpregnancy interval. *American Journal of Clinical Nutrition* (1987) 45: 29–41.

Caulfield, L., Witter, F., Stoltzfus, R. Determinants of gestational weight gain outside the recommended ranges among black and white women. *Obstetrics and Gynecology* (1996) 87 (5): 760–766.

Cnattingius, S., Bergstrom, R., et al. Prepregnancy weight and the risk of adverse pregnancy outcomes. *New England Journal of Medicine* (1998) 338 (3): 147–152.

Coustan, D., Carpenter, M., et al. Gestational diabetes: Predictors of subsequent disordered glucose metabolism. *American Journal of Obstetrics and Gynecology* (1993) 168 (4): 1139–1145.

Crowell, D. T. Weight change in the postpartum period. *Journal of Nurse Midwifery* (1995) 40 (5): 418–423.

Dacus., J., et al. Gestational diabetes: Postpartum glucose tolerance testing. *American Journal of Obstetrics and Gynecology* (1994) 171 (4): 927–931.

David, R. J., Collins, J. W., Jr. Differing birth weight among infants of U.S.-born blacks, African-American blacks, and U.S.-born whites. *New England Journal of Medicine* (1997) 337 (17): 1209–1214.

Davidson, J. A., Roberts, V. L. Gestational diabetes: Ensuring a successful outcome. *Postgraduate Medicine* (1996) 99 (3): 165–172.

DiCianni, G., Benzi, L., et al. Neonatal outcome and obstetric complications in women with gestational diabetes: Effects of maternal body mass index. *International Journal of Obesity and Related Metabolic Disorders* (1996) 20 (5): 445–449.

Dornhorst, A. Implications of gestational diabetes for the health of the mother. *British Journal of Obstetrics and Gynecology* (1994) 101: 286–290.

Dornhorst, A., Girling, J. Management of gestation diabetes mellitus. *New England Journal of Medicine* (1995) 333 (19): 1–4.

Edwards, L., Hellerstedt, W., et al. Pregnancy complications and birth outcomes in obese and normal-weight women: Effects of gestational weight change. *Obstetrics and Gynecology* (1996) 87 (3): 389–394.

Ellard, G., Johnstone, F., et al. Smoking during pregnancy: The dose dependence of birthweight deficits. *British Journal of Obstetrics and Gynecology* (1996) 103 (8): 806–813.

Foster, J. W., Jr. The enigma of low birth weight and race. *New England Journal of Medicine* (1997) 337 (17): 1232–1233.

Garner, P., Okun, N., et al. A randomized controlled trial of strict glycemic control and tertiary level obstetric care versus routine obstetric care in the management of gestational diabetes: A pilot study. *American Journal of Obstetrics and Gynecology* (1997) 1: 190–195.

Goldenberg, R. L., Rouse, D. J. Medical progress: Prevention of premature birth. *New England Journal of Medicine* (1998) 339 (5): 313–320.

Johnson, J. W. C., Yancey, M. K. A critique of the new recommendations for weight gain in pregnancy. *American Journal of Obstetrics and Gynecology* (1996) 174 (1): 254–258.

Kaufmann, R., et al. Gestational diabetes diagnostic criteria: Long-term maternal follow-up. *American Journal of Obstetrics and Gynecology* (1995) 172 (2): 621–625.

Lantz, M., Chez, R., et al. Maternal weight gain patterns and birth weight outcome in twin gestation. *Obstetrics and Gynecology* (1996) 87 (4): 551–556.

Maresh, M., Beard, R., Bray, C., et al. Factors predisposing to and outcome of gestational diabetes. *Obstetrics and Gynecology* (1989) 74: 342–346.

Parham, E., Astrom, M. F., King, S. H. The association of pregnancy weight gain with the mother's postpartum weight. *American Dietetic Association* (1990) 90 (4): 550–554.

Rossner, S., Ohlin, A. Pregnancy as a risk factor for obesity: Lessons from the Stockholm Pregnancy and Weight Development Study. *Obesity Research* (1995) 3 (suppl 2): 267S–275S.

Schauberger, C., et al. Postpartum weight loss: Factors that influence weight loss in the puerperium. *Obstetrics and Gynecology* (1992) 79: 424–428.

Siega-Riz, A., Adair, L., Hobel, C. Maternal underweight status and inadequate rate of weight gain during the third trimester of pregnancy increases the risk of preterm delivery. *Journal of Nutrition* (1996) 126 (1): 146–153.

Stanner, S. A., et al. Does malnutrition in uteri determine diabetes and coronary heart disease in adulthood? Results from the Leningrad siege study, a cross sectional study. *British Medical Journal* (1997) 315: 1342–1349.

Weeks, J., Major, C., et al. Gestational diabetes: Does the presence of risk factors influence perinatal outcome? *American Journal of Obstetrics and Gynecology* (1994) 171 (4): 1003–1007.

Weller, K. A. Diagnosis and management of gestational diabetes. *American Family Physician* (1996) 53 (6): 2053–2057.

Index

abdomen:
  fat in, 95, 96
  toning of, 112–114
acne, 94
adipose tissue, *see* fat, body
adoption, depression and, 64–65
adrenal glands, 87
African-American women:
  breast-feeding of, 138
  diabetes and, 176, 178
  married vs. single, 14
  obesity of, 13–14
age:
  breast-feeding and, 140
  diabetes and, 177
  metabolism and, 54
  postpartum weight loss and, 19
airline food, 213
alcohol, 82, 107–108
Alcott, Louisa May, 197
alternative medicine, 88–89, 144
amaranth, 84
amenorrhea, 54
American Academy of Pediatrics, 48, 126–127
American College of Obstetrics and Gynecology, 152, 180
American Diabetes Association, 180
American Heart Association, 13
American Journal of Clinical Nutrition, 136
American Psychiatric Association, 89
amino acids, 68–69, 72, 79
amniotic fluid, 50
amphetamines, 153
Angelou, Maya, 191
anorectics, 100
antidepressants, 68
antioxidants, 109, 213
anxiety, 63
appearance:
  and the real you, 20

in second postpartum trimester, 93–94
  weight loss and, 12
appetite:
  effects of HCS on, 23
  endorphins and, 56
  fad diets and, 60
  fat cells and, 97, 99, 100
  hormones and, 10, 21, 23, 26, 28, 29, 53, 54, 55, 94, 97–100, 102, 132–134
  neurotransmitters and, 22, 61
  pregnancy and, 23, 26, 28, 53
  spicy foods and, 215
  stimulation of, 94, 132–134, 195, 201
  suppression of, 10, 28, 29, 30, 53, 54, 60, 215
appetizers, 207
apples, 205
applesauce, 191
Arby's, 251
Aristotle, 203
asparagus, 201
asthma, 106, 213
atherosclerosis (hardening of the arteries), 74, 104
attitude makeover, 10–11
avocados, 211, 215

babies, 64, 203
  average weight of, 50
  back-saver plan for picking up, 91
  benefits of breast-feeding to, 127–128, 135
  effects of gestational diabetes on, 178–179
  effects of postpartum depression on, 65
  health risks of overweight to, 161–162
  low birth weight, 152, 153, 160
  World War II food problems and, 152–153
baby blahs, 66–67, 68
  symptoms of, 66
baby blues, 61–65
  of E.M., 63
  risk factors for, 63, 64

Index